**Official Journal of the Internationa... ...
Blood Purification**

Blood Purification

Founded 1983; edited by K. Schaefer (1983–1988)

KARGER

Printed in Switzerland
on acid-free paper by
Thür AG Offsetdruck, Pratteln

Appears bimonthly:
1 volume per year (6 issues)

Submission: Only original papers written in English are considered and should be sent to:

S. Karger AG
Editorial Dept. 'Blood Purification'
P.O. Box
CH-4009 Basel (Switzerland)

Manuscripts should be submitted in quadruplicate (with four sets of illustrations of which one is an original), typewritten double-spaced on one side of the paper, with a wide margin.

Conditions: All manuscripts are subject to editorial review. Manuscripts are received with the explicit understanding that they are not under simultaneous consideration by any other publication. Submission of an article for publication implies the transfer of the copyright from the author to the publisher upon acceptance. Accepted papers become the permanent property of 'Blood Purification' and may not be reproduced by any means, in whole or in part, without the written consent of the publisher. It is the author's responsibility to obtain permission to reproduce illustrations, tables, etc. from other publications.

Arrangement:
Title page: The first page of each paper should indicate the title (main title underlined), the authors' names, and the institute where the work was conducted. A short title for use as running head as well as the full address of the author to whom correspondence should be sent are also required.
Full address: The exact postal address complete with postal code must be given at the bottom of the title page. Please also supply Phone, Fax, and E-mail numbers.
Key words: For indexing purposes, a list of 3–10 key words in English is essential.
Abstract: Each paper needs an abstract of up to 10 lines.
Small type: Paragraphs which can or must be set in smaller type (case histories, test methods, etc.) should be indicated with a 'p' (petit) in the margin on the left-hand side.
Footnotes: Avoid footnotes. When essential, they are numbered consecutively and typed at the foot of the appropriate page.
Tables and illustrations: Tables and illustrations (both numbered in Arabic numerals) should be prepared on separate sheets. Tables require a heading and figures a legend, also prepared on a separate sheet. For the reproduction of illustrations, only good drawings and original photographs can be accepted; negatives or photocopies cannot be used. Due to technical reasons, figures with a screen background should not be submitted. When possible, group several illustrations on one block for reproduction (max. size 140 × 188 mm) or provide crop marks. On the back of each illustration, indicate its number, the author's name, and 'top' with a soft pencil.

Color illustrations: Up to 6 color illustrations per page can now be integrated with the text at the reduced price of CHF 600.– / USD 545.00 per page. Color illustrations are reproduced at the author's expense.

References: In the text identify references by Arabic numerals [in square brackets]. Material submitted for publication but not yet accepted should be noted as 'unpublished data' and not be included in the reference list. The list of references should include only those publications which are cited in the text. Do not alphabetize; number references in the order in which they are first mentioned in the text. The surnames of the authors followed by initials should be given. There should be no punctuation other than a comma to separate the authors. Cite all authors, 'et al' is not sufficient. Abbreviate journal names according to the Index Medicus system. (Also see International Committee of Medical Journal Editors: Uniform requirements for manuscripts submitted to biomedical journals. Br Med J 1988;296: 401–405.)
Examples
(a) Papers published in periodicals: Kauffman HF, van der Heide S, Beaumont F, Blok H, de Vries K: Class-specific antibody determination against *Aspergillus fumigatus* by means of the enzyme-linked immunosorbent assay. III. Comparative study: IgG, IgA, IgM ELISA titers, precipitating antibodies and IgE binding after fractionation of the antigen. Int Arch Allergy Appl Immunol 1986;80:300–306.
(b) Monographs: Matthews DE, Farewell VT: Using and Understanding Medical Statistics. Basel, Karger, 1985.
(c) Edited books: Hardy WD Jr, Essex M: FeLV-induced feline acquired immune deficiency syndrome: A model for human AIDS; in Klein E (ed): Acquired Immunodeficiency Syndrome. Prog Allergy. Basel, Karger, 1986, vol 37, pp 353–376.
Further details: Authors may consult our leaflet 'Rules for the Preparation of Manuscripts', available on request from the Publisher, S. Karger AG, P.O. Box, CH-4009 Basel (Switzerland).

Rapid communication: Manuscripts intended for rapid communication must present new findings of sufficient importance to justify their accelerated acceptance. They should follow the general arrangement of research papers except that the separate sections should not be formally titled. They should not be more than three pages in length (including figures, tables and references). Proofs are checked by the Managing Editor and not sent to the authors. Review will be rapid, and once accepted, the paper will be included in the next planned issue.

Page charges: There is no page charge for papers of 4 or fewer printed pages (including tables, illustrations and references). Each additional complete or partial page is charged to the author at CHF 245.– / USD 196.00. The allotted size of a paper is equal to approx. 7 manuscript pages (including tables, illustrations and references).

Galley proofs: Unless indicated otherwise, galley proofs are sent to the first-named author and should be returned with the least possible delay. Alterations made in galley proofs, other than the correction of printer's errors, are charged to the author. No page proofs are supplied.

Reprints: Order forms and a price list are sent with the galley proofs. Orders submitted after the issue is printed are subject to considerably higher prices. Allow five weeks from date of publication for delivery of reprints.

KARGER
E-Mail karger@karger.ch
Fax +41 61 306 12 34
http://www.karger.ch

General Information
http://www.karger.ch/journals/bpu/bpudes.htm

Blood Purification

Publication data: 'Blood Purification' is published 6 times annually. Volume 14 with 6 issues appears in 1996.

Subscription rates: Subscriptions run for a full calendar year. Prices are given per volume.

Personal subscription:

Subscription	+ *postage and handling*
CHF 275.40	+ CHF 22.10 Europe
CHF 275.40	+ CHF 33.60 Overseas
USD 211.80	+ USD 22.10

(Must be in the name of, billed to, and paid by an individual. Order must be marked 'personal subscription'.)

Institutional subscription:

Subscription	+ *postage and handling*
CHF 459.–	+ CHF 27.60 Europe
CHF 459.–	+ CHF 42.– Overseas
USD 353.00	+ USD 27.60

Airmail postage: CHF 36.–, USD 30.00. (Extra per volume.)

Discount subscription prices:
International Society of Blood Purification

Microforms: Please direct all enquiries and orders to:
University Microfilms Inc.
300 North Zeeb Road, P.O. Box 1346
Ann Arbor, MI 48106-1346 (USA)

Subscription orders: Orders can be placed at agencies, bookstores, directly with the Publisher S. Karger AG, P.O. Box, CH – 4009 Basel (Switzerland) or with any of the following distributors:

Deutschland: S. Karger GmbH, Postfach
D – 79095 Freiburg

France: Librairie Luginbühl
36, bd de Latour-Maubourg
F–75007 Paris

Great Britain, Ireland: S. Karger Publishers
11 Ravenscroft Road
Beckenham, Kent BR3 4TP

USA: S. Karger Publishers, Inc.
26 West Avon Road, P.O. Box 529
Farmington, CT 06085

India, Bangladesh, Sri Lanka:
S. Karger India Subscription Agency
B – 5/132 Safdarjung Enclave
New Delhi-110029

Japan: Katakura Libri, Inc.
Take 1 Bldg, 2nd Floor
4-5-7 Yushima, Bunkyo-ku
Tokyo 113

Change of address: Both old and new address should be sent to the subscription source.

Single issues and back volumes: Information can be obtained through the Publisher.

Advertising: Correspondence and rate requests should be addressed to the Publisher.

Bibliographic indices: This journal is regularly listed in bibliographic services, including *Current Contents*®.

Book Reviews: Books are accepted for review by special agreement.

Guidelines for Disk Submission

Karger Publishers welcomes the submission of manuscripts on disk.
Please observe the 'Instructions to Authors' as well as the following guidelines:

Technical Data

Storage medium is a 3.5- or 5.25-inch disk.
The preferred word processing package is Word for Windows®. Other commonly used PC text programs are also accepted, as well as ASCII formats.
MacIntosh® is also acceptable. However **1.44 Byte HD** in ASCII is preferred.

Handling

All manuscripts accepted for Karger publications are subject to copy-editing. It is therefore essential that you send us a **double-spaced printout** of your manuscript which exactly matches the disk.

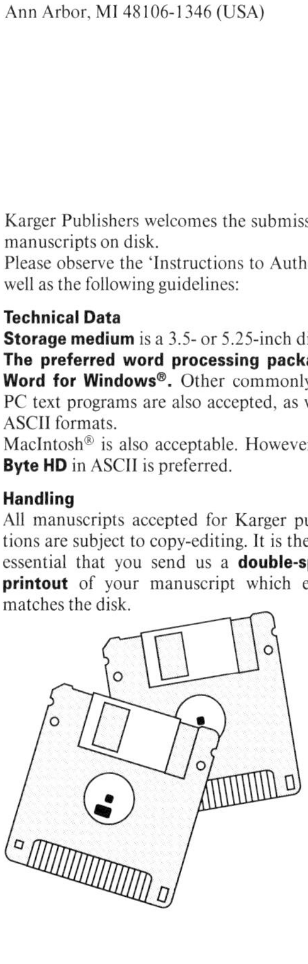

Any subsequent revised versions should be clearly marked as such, both on the disk and on the manuscript.
The copy-edited manuscript and the disk will be returned to you along with the galley proofs. Please be sure to **check the galleys against the manuscript** in which changes introduced by the copy-editor and/or questions will be marked.
Please **label** your disk with (a) the title of the journal or book for which it is submitted, (b) a short version of the paper title, (c) your name, (d) the software and hardware used and (e) the file names contained.
Do not place more than one article in a file.

Text Arrangement

Please follow the general rules about style given in the 'Instructions to Authors' or 'Rules for the Preparation of Manuscripts'.
Be sure to use the same type style for headings of the same ranking throughout the text. Be consistent and stick to the same work pattern throughout the manuscript.
Do not use automatic page numbering. Number the pages by hand.
Text and headings should be ranged left throughout, without word breaks. **Do not center, space, or use block letters** for text and headings (except for abbreviations). Do not split words (neither by hand nor automatically).
Do not use indentations anywhere in the manuscript, including the references. To mark the beginning of a paragraph, leave one blank line between paragraphs. Do not use a hyphenating program. Use the possibilities of your text program to emphasize text parts, e.g. **Bold,** *Italic,* $_{\text{Sub-}}$ and ^{Superscript}.
Insert one (and only one) space after each interpunctuation mark – e.g. at the end of sentences and with reference numbers, i.e. [22, 27, 35].
When using **special characters** not available on a standard keyboard (including Greek characters) please do so by a readily identifiable code, and use the same code throughout the manuscript. Supply a **complete list of the codes used** at the beginning of the text or include a 'Read-me-file'.
Do not use spaces in tables; use the tabulator. Operation data within tables (e.g. 15.1 ± 7.23) should be formatted in one column, not split into two.
Illustrations and mathematical formulae will be handled conventionally.

KARGER
E-Mail karger@karger.ch
Fax + 41 61 306 12 34
http://www.karger.ch

Selected Presentations from the Joint Annual Meeting of the RPA-NIDDK 1995

Guest Editors
Thomas A. Golper, Little Rock, Ark.
M. James Scherbenske, Bethesda, Md.

9 figures and 18 tables, 1996

KARGER

S. Karger
Medical and Scientific Publishers
Basel · Freiburg · Paris · London
New York · New Delhi · Bangkok
Singapore · Tokyo · Sydney

Drug Dosage
The authors and the publisher have exerted every effort to ensure that drug selection and dosage set forth in this text are in accord with current recommendations and practice at the time of publication. However, in view of ongoing research, changes in government regulations, and the constant flow of information relating to drug therapy and drug reactions, the reader is urged to check the package insert for each drug for any change in indications and dosage and for added warnings and precautions. This is particularly important when the recommended agent is a new and/or infrequently employed drug.

Printed in Switzerland on acid-free paper by
Thür AG Offsetdruck, Pratteln
ISBN 3-8055-6371-X

Blood Purification

Vol. 14, No. 4, 1996

Contents

KARGER

E-Mail karger@karger.ch
Fax + 41 61 306 12 34
http://www.karger.ch

The list of contents is available at:
http://www.karger.ch/journals/bpu/bpucont.htm

Blood Purification

Preface

Lee W. Henderson

The NIDDK/RPA meeting had two major themes which are presented in this issue of *Blood Purification.*

Ethic and/or minority groups suffer an inordinately high rate of renal disease and its complications. This has important ramifications for world-wide health. Sociocultural vs. genetic explanations are raised in the context of hypertension, diabetes, malnutrition, acidosis, and immunologic function. Groups discussed include Afro-Americans, Native Americans (Indians), and Hispanics. The reader will find far-reaching implications in these papers.

The second theme is hypertension/vascular disease in the ESRD setting. Are we not diagnosing (and therefore not treating) reversible renovascular disease? I am disturbed by the data of Textor and the way I manage ESRD patients. This is a clear eye-opener. The St. John's group continues to piece together cardiac hypertrophy, LV failure and ischemia picture. This, of course, leads to how aggressive should we be in our treatment of hypertension in ESRD patients, which is addressed by Dr. Rosansky.

These themes and papers are timely.

KARGER
E-Mail karger@karger.ch
Fax + 41 61 306 12 34
http://www.karger.ch

Blood Purification

Blood Purif 1996;14:278–285

William F. Owen, Jr.

Division of Nephrology,
Brigham and Women's Hospital,
and Department of Medicine,
Harvard Medical School,
Boston, Mass., USA

Racial Differences in Incidence, Outcome, and Quality of Life for African-Americans on Hemodialysis

Key Words

African-Americans, end-stage renal disease
Diabetes
Hemodialysis
Hypertension
Survival, end-stage renal disease

Abstract

African-Americans are the fastest growing racial minority with end-stage renal disease (ESRD) in the United States. Although comprising <15% of the US population, African-Americans comprise ~31% of the ESRD population. African-Americans are approximately 7 years younger than their white counterparts with ESRD. Surprisingly, although African-Americans systematically receive less dialysis than whites, their survival with ESRD is greatly improved. This improved survival with ESRD is accompanied by an improved quality of life for African-Americans. In this review, we will examine the reasons why African-Americans have an excessive incidence of selective diseases that culminate in ESRD. Furthermore, we will judge several hypotheses that may account for the improved survival enjoyed by African-Americans with ESRD. We contend that research targeted to clarify the basis for these differences between African-Americans and whites with ESRD will improve the outcomes for both populations.

'Dr. Owen, ain't it nothing but black folks on dialysis?'
R.H., 1992

Although the consequences of end-stage renal disease (ESRD) are suffered by all racial and ethnic groups, the African-American community has shouldered a disproportionate burden from this malady. Although the direct medical consequences and costs of care for ESRD are the most simply characterized of ESRD in the African-American community, it should be realized that the low rehabilitation rate of all ESRD patients has a particularly devastating consequence for the minority community. Because most African-Ameri-

KARGER

E-Mail karger@karger.ch
Fax +41 61 306 12 34
http://www.karger.ch

0253–5068/96/0144–0278$10.00/0

William F. Owen, Jr., MD
Division of Nephrology
Brigham and Women's Hospital
75 Francis Street
Boston, MA 02115 (USA)

cans live in areas that are racially segregated, the geographic predilection of ESRD is likewise segregated. Thus, the deleterious financial consequences of ESRD are particularly felt in communities and within health care systems that can least afford or can least accommodate such a costly illness. The impact of ESRD in the African-American community drains lives and resources from those it afflicts and from their community of residence. Thus the remark by R.H. is particularly poignant and summarizes the impressions of many patients of color.

Although R.H.'s impression is inaccurate, there are a disproportionate percentage of African-Americans being treated for ESRD. Although African-Americans comprise only 13% of the population of the United States, 30.8% of the ESRD population was African-American in 1991 (prevalence of 2,298 per million) [1]. The median age for African-Americans with treated ESRD is younger than for whites (57.7 and 63.7 years, respectively, for 1989–1991). Thus, African-Americans are the largest and youngest racial minority with treated ESRD. Like the entire ESRD population, the number of Medicare-eligible African-American patients has increased steadily from 12,488 in 1978 to 56,508 in 1991 [1]. The age-, sex-, and renal-diagnosis-adjusted prevalence rate of treated ESRD in African-Americans is three times that of whites (1,409 and 467 per million, respectively) [2].

Incidence and Prevalence of Selected Etiologies of ESRD

The prevalence rate of ESRD secondary to hypertension, diabetes mellitus, and glomerulonephritis is higher in African-Americans than in whites. The age- and gender-adjusted prevalence rates of hypertensive ESRD were 624 and 63 cases per million in 1988 for African-Americans and whites, respectively; diabetes mellitus was 364 and 87 cases per million, respectively, and glomerulonephritis was 224 and 97 cases per million, respectively [2]. Most of the excessive prevalence of ESRD for African-Americans is a consequence of a greatly increased incidence rate of ESRD, particularly secondary to essential hypertension, diabetes mellitus, and glomerulonephritis. A lesser contributant for the excessive prevalence of ESRD among African-Americans is their increased survival on dialysis in comparison to whites [3]. This issue is discussed in greater detail in a later section.

The most frequent diagnosed etiology for ESRD in African-Americans is hypertension. The age- and gender-adjusted rate of hypertensive ESRD is sixfold greater in African-Americans than in whites (217 and 36 per million in 1989–1991, respectively) [1]. The incidence rate for hypertensive ESRD has increased annually for both African-Americans and whites, but, surprisingly, the increase has been greatest for whites. Therefore, the percentage of African-Americans in the total population of patients with hypertensive ESRD (African-American plus white incidence of hypertensive ESRD) has declined (from 48 to 41% of all cases during 1977–1988) [4]. Nevertheless, this is still an impressive figure, especially in the light of the minority population status of African-Americans. For both African-Americans and whites, the hypertensive ESRD population has increased in age from 1977 to 1988, but the median age of African-Americans is a decade less than in whites (60 and 70 years old, respectively) [4]. Thus, in summary, in comparison to whites, African-Americans are at increased risk to develop ESRD from hypertension, especially at a younger age.

The age- and gender-adjusted incidence rate of ESRD from diabetes mellitus is 3.7-

fold greater in African-Americans than in whites (187 and 49 per million in 1989–1991, respectively) [1]. The age-specific incidence rate of diabetic ESRD in African-Americans is bimodal (peaks at age ranges 25–29 and 60–64 years) corresponding to the peak ages for type 1 and type 2 diabetes mellitus, respectively [5]. Even adjusting for the increased prevalence of diabetes mellitus in African-Americans, most ESRD occurs in association with type 2 diabetes mellitus (77%), whereas most whites develop diabetic ESRD from type 1 diabetes (58%). For both African-Americans and whites, the risk of diabetic ESRD over 10 years is greater for type 1 than for type 2 diabetes (African-Americans plus whites 5.82 vs. 0.5%, respectively) [5]. However, in directly comparing African-Americans and whites with type 2 diabetes mellitus, the probability of developing ESRD over a decade is fourfold greater for African-Americans. Because of the increased numbers of African-Americans with type 2 versus type 1 diabetes mellitus, most cases of diabetic ESRD in African-Americans are secondary to type 2 diabetes. Thus, in summary, in comparison to whites, African-Americans are at increased risk of diabetic ESRD, especially from type 2 diabetes mellitus.

Lastly, glomerulonephritides, such as focal and segmental glomerulosclerosis, membranous nephropathy, membranoproliferative glomerulonephritis, and Goodpasture's syndrome, are treated at higher incidence rates in African-Americans than in whites (49 and 19 per million in 1989–1991, respectively) [1]. However, it must be realized that diagnostic misclassification may be a significant problem for analysis of glomerulonephritides that result in ESRD, because of the absence of either simple or standardized diagnostic criteria. An increased incidence and prevalence of disorders associated with glomerulonephritis, such as heroin nephropathy and human immunodeficiency virus (HIV) nephropathy, may explain some of the increased incidence rate among African-Americans [6]. However, it appears that the deleterious nephrologic course of selected glomerular disorders, such as HIV infections, is accelerated in African-Americans.

Potential Factors Contributing to Observed Racial Differences in ESRD

The observed differences in the incidence rate for ESRD between African-Americans and whites may be accounted for by at least two different explanations. The first of these is a disease-specific model that assumes that the progression of renal disease to ESRD is no different between African-Americans and whites; but the increased prevalence rate in African-Americans is the result of their exaggerated incidence rate. The alternative model is a race-specific model that supposes that indifferent of the type of renal disease, its progression to ESRD is enhanced among African-Americans. The race-specific model may be further segregated into two categories. The genetic model argues that genetic differences between African-Americans and whites result in increased susceptibility to the pathobiologic processes that culminate in ESRD or a diminished response to therapies that attenuate the progression to ESRD. A demographic model suggests that race is a surrogate for deleterious socioeconomic variables and that the apparent race-related increase in susceptibility to ESRD is a consequence of a psychosocial environment that limits access to health care and medications and tolerates deleterious health-related behavior.

The socioeconomic barriers to adequate health care for African-Americans are formidable. With unemployment being approximately threefold greater in African-American than white households and approximately 30% of African-Americans living below the poverty level, it is unsurprising that their access to medical care is compromised. An example of such is that 40% of African-American births occur without prenatal care being delivered until the second half of the pregnancy [7]. Suggestive evidence that a low household income may be a risk factor for ESRD is the observed inverse correlation between household income and the prevalence of ESRD [7]. Similarly, using the United States Renal Data System, a strong and inverse correlation was found between income and incidence of ESRD for African-Americans and whites, especially for African-Americans [8].

Insufficient data exist to support either the diesase-specific model or the race-specific model alone. Instead, the increased incidence of ESRD among African-Americans seems to be a consequence of the interaction of both of these variables. An example of the interplay of these factors for hypertensive ESRD is provided by the prospective analysis of the incidence of hypertensive ESRD in the Maryland Regional ESRD Registry (ESRD Network 31) [9]. In a univariate analysis, the authors reported that hypertensive ESRD was statistically associated with African-American race (relative risk 5.6), prevalence of hypertension (1.78) and its severity (1.72), diabetes mellitus (1.58), and adverse socioeconomic environment (relative risk 2.53–4.27). However, even after using a multivariate model that included race, prevalence, and severity of hypertension, diabetes mellitus, and socioeconomic status, African-Americans persisted in having a relative risk for the development of ESRD of 4.5. Therefore, despite increased exposure to factors that predispose African-Americans to the development of hypertensive ESRD, these well-recognized risk factors alone cannot completely account for the increased odds risk of renal failure.

Risk factor analyses such as this suggest that African-Americans may be genetically more susceptible to hypertensive ESRD. Support for this hypothesis is provided from an analysis of the hypertensive participants of the Multiple Risk Factor Intervention Trial (MRFIT) [10]. African-American and white male patients with mild to moderate hypertension (diastolic blood pressure >90 mm Hg) and normal renal function were treated with the same level of effectiveness by year 2 of the study (diastolic blood pressures <85 mm Hg). Whereas whites had a decrease in serum creatinine during the 7-year period of the study, African-Americans had a significant increment in their serum creatinine level (+0.035 mg/dl). Thus, this level of blood pressure reduction did not protect African-Americans from hypertensive renal disease. Similarly, another analysis of treated essential hypertension found that sustained antihypertensive control (mean diastolic blood pressure ≤ 90 mm Hg) did not prevent a decline in renal function, especially in African-Americans [11]. The African-American participants were twice as likely as whites to undergo a significant increment in their serum creatinine concentration. Although race alone was a significant independent risk factor for progressive renal insufficiency, a stepwise regression analysis with backwards elimination of significant variables revealed that the African-Americans with progressive renal insufficiency were also more likely to have missed office visits and be of a lower socioeconomic class.

Similarly, for diabetes mellitus, the increased incidence rate of ESRD in African-Americans is not a simple consequence of an increased prevalence of diabetes. Using data from a population-based ecological study, a univariate analysis found that the relative risk of ESRD secondary to diabetes was increased for race (African-American 3.42), prevalence of diabetes mellitus (2.35), hypertension

(1.65), socioeconomic status (1.28), and lack of health insurance (1.98) [12]. A subsequent multivariate analysis using all variables except race revealed that African-Americans had a 4.8-fold relative risk of ESRD secondary to type 2 diabetes mellitus, but no excessive risk as compared with whites for type 1 diabetes mellitus. Thus, an etiologic interplay between race and socioeconomic status is suggested for hypertensive ESRD and diabetic ESRD, not simply an increased prevalence of hypertension and diabetes mellitus, respectively.

Recently, a fascinating hypothesis has been proposed that may account for the interaction between genetic susceptibility to ESRD and adverse socioeconomic circumstances. Entitled the 'low-birth-weight hypothesis', this theory is based on observations of the consequences of low birth weight on kidney and pancreatic function post partum [13]. In animals, low birth weight may be casually associated with a nephron deficit that is never recovered and may be of sufficient severity to contribute to the development of glomerulosclerosis with hypertension. A low birth weight is also associated with structural abnormalities of the endocrine pancreas such as a diminished number of β-cells and a decreased vasculature to the Islets of Langerhans. Epidemiological support for a correlation between low birth weight in humans and the development of hypertension and diabetes mellitus is provided by the observation of a statistically significant inverse correlation between birth weight and systolic blood pressure and incidence rate of type 2 diabetes mellitus. Moderate low birth weight infants (1.5–2.5 kg) are much more common among African-American than white women (9.3/100 and 4/100 live births, respectively). Arguably, low birth weight is a major contributory factor towards the development of hypertension and type 2 diabetes mellitus because of its causal association with oligonephropathy and pancreatic dysgenesis, respectively. Furthermore, in that many of the same socioeconomic deficiencies that give rise to low birth weight are risk factors for the later development of ESRD secondary to hypertension and diabetes mellitus, this theory is especially plausible.

However, the absolute contribution of low birth weight to the excessive incidence rates of ESRD among African-Americans is unclear. The interaction between genetic and socioeconomic factors is certainly much more complex than the pathobiologic scheme outlined by the low-birth-weight hypothesis. For example, in an analysis of the correlation between blood pressure, skin color, and socioeconomic status among African-Americans, it was observed that blood pressures were correlated to darker skin color only for those blacks of a lower socioeconomic status [14]. Although these data are compatible with the genetic linkage of hypertensive loci with genes conferring a darker skin color, they are also in agreement with the concept of 'John Henryism' – darker colored African-Americans of a lower socioeconomic status are exposed to greater psychosocial stress reflected in higher blood pressures.

Survival of African-Americans with ESRD

African-Americans with ESRD have better survivals than whites, even after adjustments for gender and age and after transplant recipients have been excluded [3]. Whites have a 29% higher risk of death than African-Americans that is accounted for by their increased risk of death, especially secondary to cardiac events, withdrawal from dialysis, and infections. Despite knowledge of the cause of death, the basis of the improved survival for

African-Americans is unclear. Potential explanations include: (1) the selection of healthier African-Americans for dialysis treatments; (2) misdiagnosis of the etiology of ESRD among African-Americans; (3) enhanced delivery of dialysis to African-Americans; (4) improved nutrition among African-Americans, and (5) enhanced quality of life.

Selection of Healthier African-Americans for Dialysis Treatments

In the American population at large, the age- and gender-adjusted death rate for African-Americans versus whites between the ages of 35–77 years is 32% higher for African-Americans. A revealing insight into the potential role of competing risks is provided in a population analysis of six common risk factors for early death (smoking, hypertension, hypercholesterolemia, alcohol consumption, obesity, and diabetes mellitus) [15]. For African-Americans 35–54 years old, approximately 30% of their excessive risk could be accounted for by the six risk factors and another third by family income. The remaining third was statistically unexplained. In contrast, African-Americans 55–77 years old experienced no increased mortality in comparison to whites. After 77 years old, African-Americans enjoy improved survival in comparison to whites. One explanation of this phenomenon is that increased risk factor exposure among African-Americans results in their early demise, leaving a surviving group with a low mortality risk. A similar process may be operational among the ESRD populations, such that those whites that develop ESRD have greater risk factor exposure for mortality than African-Americans. Alternatively, an unconscious selection bias may exist such that African-Americans that are selected for maintenance dialysis have fewer risk factors than whites. Neither of these theories has been formally evaluated.

Misclassification of the Etiology of ESRD among African-Americans

Diseases like hypertension and diabetes mellitus may either cause renal failure, contribute to the demise of renal failure from another etiology, or, in the case of hypertension, be a consequence of the renal failure. Reporting bias may be especially problematic for African-American patients who often present to the nephrologist with advanced states of renal disease such that the proceeding nephrologic history and signs are unavailable. In the case of hypertension, 40% of the African-American patients with 'hypertensive ESRD' in the Watts/Willowbrook area of Los Angeles have had hypertension for <5 years on average, but have used recreational drugs like crack cocaine [16]. Similar diagnostic uncertainty exists in the case of diabetes mellitus. In a case-controlled study, the percentage of African-Americans with ESRD secondary to diabetes mellitus was 41% using the population-attributable risks: (incidence of ESRD in the entire population – incidence of ESRD among patients without diabetes) ÷ incidence of ESRD in the entire population. In contrast, using their clinical diagnosis, only 29% of the sample had diabetic ESRD. For whites, this diagnostic discrepancy did not exist. Thus, it is possible that African-Americans with ESRD secondary to diseases associated with an improved clinical outcome have been misdiagnosed. The resultant disease-adjusted analysis of outcome would be skewed. There are no data to support this hypothesis.

Enhanced Quantity of Dialysis Delivered to African-Americans

Because the quantity of delivered dialysis is a major predictor of outcome for patients with ESRD, arguably African-Americans may receive greater quantities of dialysis than whites. However, this has recently been demonstrated to not be correct. Regionally, even after adjustment for a greater weight for African-American patients, their Kt/V was significantly lower than that of whites (1.05 and 1.18, respectively) [17]. Nationally, 36% of the African-Americans and 46% of the whites with ESRD received urea reduction ratios of ≥ 65% [18]. Large geographic variations exist in delivered dialysis such that those regions of the country that contained the largest number of African-American patients were often the areas with the lowest percentage of patients with urea reduction ratios ≥ 65%. Therefore, differences in dialysis adequacy do not explain the survival advantage enjoyed by African-Americans.

Improved Nutrition among African-Americans

Using a large data base that captures information on patient demographics, outcomes, and common laboratory test results, previous analyses have demonstrated that surrogates of nutrition are powerful predictors of outcome for patients maintained on hemodialysis (serum albumin and creatinine concentrations) [19, 20]. Higher albumin and creatinine concentrations are predictive of better patient survival. Similarly, statistical models were generated to analyze the odds risk of death based on patient case mix variables alone. The odds risk of death associated with white race in comparison to African-Americans was observed to be 1.42 [21]. The potential laboratory predictors of outcome were then added to a logistic regression model in a stepwise manner, and their effects on the case mix variable were observed. The addition of the laboratory variable to the logistic regression model reduced the relative risk of death from being white to 1.09. Specifically, the serum creatinine concentration was the laboratory variable that accounted for this reduction in risk. In that the creatinine generation rate reflects somatic protein content, this biologic link most likely is derived from the patients' nutritional status. Similarly, obese patients have a lower mortality with ESRD, and African-Americans suffer a higher prevalence of obesity [22]. All of these data suggest that African-Americans have an enhanced nutritional status that ascribes them with a survival advantage to whites with ESRD.

African-Americans Have a Better Quality of Life with ESRD

Arguably, the best measure of a dialysis patient's quality of life is the willingness to continue dialysis treatments. Alternatively, patients that are extremely dissatisfied with their life will die prematurely by discontinuing dialysis. African-Americans voluntarily discontinue dialysis treatments with far less frequency than whites (white:black death risk ratio 2.72) [3]. Arguably, increased dissatisfaction with maintenance dialysis by whites may be manifest as medical noncompliance towards other components of the dialysis treatment or the acquisition of deleterious health-related behaviors that would affect their survival. This theory has not been examined.

Conclusions

The impact of ESRD within the African-American community is legion. Most African-Americans either know someone or have a relative who requires maintenance dialysis. We often describe the 'graying' of America's ESRD Program to convey the increasing age of its subscribers. Continuing with this analogy, we must not forget the 'browning' of the ESRD Program, as posed by RH's question.

References

1 US Renal Data System, USRDS 1994 Annual Data Report. Bethesda, National Institutes of Health, National Institute of Diabetes and Digestive and Kidney Diseases, August 1994.
2 Feldman HI, Klag MJ, Chiapella AP, Whelton PK: End-stage renal disease in US minority groups. Am J Kidney Dis 1992;14:397–410.
3 Bloembergen WE, Port FK, Mauger EA, Wolfe RA: Causes of death in dialysis patients: Racial and gender differences. J Am Soc Nephrol 1994; 5:1231–1242.
4 USRDS 1992 Annual Data Report: Mortality of blacks and whites with end-stage renal disease attributed to hypertension. Am J Kidney Dis 1992;20:27–31.
5 Cowie CC, Port FK, Wolfe RA, Savage PJ, Moll PP, Hawthorne VM: Disparities in incidence of diabetic end-stage renal disease according to race and type of diabetes. N Engl J Med 1989;321:1074–1079.
6 Smith SR, Svetkey LP, Dennis VW: Racial differences in the incidence and progression of renal disease. Kidney Int 1991;40:815–822.
7 Rostand SG: US minority groups and end-stage renal disease: A disproportionate share. Am J Kidney Dis 1992;19:411–413.
8 Young EW, Mauger EA, Jiang K-H, Port FK, Wolfe RA: Socioeconomic status and end-stage renal disease in the United States. Kidney Int 1994; 45:907–911.
9 Whittle JC, Whelton PK, Seideler AJ, Klag MJ: Does racial variation in risk factors explain black-white differences in the incidence of hypertensive renal disease. Arch Intern Med 1991;151:1359–1364.
10 Walker WG, Neaton JD, Cutler JA, Neuwirth R, Cohen JD, MRFIT Research Group: Renal function change in hypertensive members of the Multiple Risk Factor Intervention Trial. JAMA 1992;268:3085–3091.
11 Rostand SG; Brown G, Kirk KA, Rutsky EA, Dustan HP: Renal insufficiency in treated hypertension. N Engl J Med 1989;320:684–688.
12 Brancati FL, Whittle JC, Whelton PK, Seidler AJ, Klag MJ: The excess incidence of diabetic end-stage renal disease among blacks: A population-based study of potential explanatory factors. JAMA 1992;268:3079–3084.
13 Lopes AAS, Port FK: The low birth weight hypothesis as a plausible explanation for the black/white differences in hypertension, non-insulin-dependent diabetes, and end-stage renal disease. Am J Kidney Dis 1995;25:350–356.
14 Klag MJ, Whelton PK, Coresh J, Grim LE, Kuller LH: The association of skin color with blood pressure in US blacks with low socioeconomic status. JAMA 1991;265:599–603.
15 Otten MW, Teutsch SM, Williamson DF, Marks JS: The effect of known risk factors on the excess mortality of black adults in the United States. JAMA 1990;263: 845–851.
16 Thornhill-Joynes M, Norris KC, Witana SC, Ward HJ, Barbour B: The impact of substance abuse on hypertensive end-stage renal disease in inner city African-Americans (abstract). J Am Soc Nephrol 1994;5: 342.
17 Sherman RA, Cody RP, Solanchick JC: Racial differences in the delivery of dialysis. Am J Kidney Dis 1993;21:632–634.
18 1994 ESRD Core Indicators Project: Initial Results. Baltimore, Md., Department of Health and Human Services, Health Care Financing Administration, Health Standards and Quality Bureau, 1994.
19 Lowrie EG, Lew NL: Death risk in hemodialysis patients: The predictive value of commonly measured variables and an evaluation of death rate differences between facilities. Am J Kidney Dis 1990;15;458–482.
20 Owen WF, Lew NL, Lui Y, Lowrie EG, Lazarus JM: The urea reduction ratio and serum albumin concentration as predictors of mortality in patients undergoing hemodialysis. N Engl J Med 1993;329:1001–1006.
21 Lowrie EG, Lew NL, Huang WH: Race and diabetes as death risk predictors in hemodialysis patients. Kidney Int 1992;42(suppl 38):22–31.
22 US Renal Data System, USRDS 1992 Annual Data Report: Comorbid conditions and correlations with mortality risk among 3,399 incident hemodialysis patients. Am J Kidney Dis 1992;20(suppl):32–38.

Blood Purification

Blood Purif 1996;14:286–292

Jacqueline A. Pugh

Mexican-American Medical Treatment Effectiveness Center, Department of Medicine, Division of General Medicine, University of Texas Health Science Center at San Antonio, and
Audie L. Murphy Memorial Veterans Hospital, San Antonio, Tex., USA

Diabetic Nephropathy and End-Stage Renal Disease in Mexican Americans

Key Words
End-stage renal disease
Diabetes mellitus
Mexican American diabetic nephropathy

Abstract
Hispanics are the second largest minority group in the United States. Mexican Americans (MAs) are the largest subgroup at 14 million in 1990. MAs have a two- to threefold increased prevalence of non-insulin-dependent diabetes mellitus. Population-based studies of MAs with non-insulin-dependent diabetes have shown that these patients may be more likely than non-Hispanic whites to develop proteinuria and are more likely to develop end-stage renal disease. The reasons for this excess risk are yet to be completely elucidated, but may be due to worse glycemic control, worse blood pressure control when hypertension does occur, worse access to medical care, and/or genetics. When MAs are treated for diabetic end-stage renal disease, they have better survival. Much less data are available for other Hispanic subgroups. From a public health perspective, higher incidence and longer survival as well as a relatively young and rapidly growing population predict an increasing burden for MAs if prevention measures are not instituted soon.

Hispanics are the second largest minority group in the United States. Mexican Americans are the largest subgroup at 14 million in 1990 and are growing at a faster rate than the rest of the population. The majority of Mexican Americans live in Texas and California. Mexican Americans have both increased prevalence (2- to 3-fold) [1–3] and incidence of non-insulin-dependent diabetes mellitus (NIDDM) [4, 5], thought secondary to their Native American genetic admixture. Studies are now addressing whether the rate of complications observed among Mexican Americans is excessive after adjusting for their higher rates of NIDDM.

KARGER

E-Mail karger@karger.ch
Fax + 41 61 306 12 34
http://www.karger.ch

Jacqueline A. Pugh, MD
Audie L. Murphy Memorial Veterans Hospital
Ambulatory Care 11C6
7400 Merton Minter Blvd.
San Antonio, TX 78284 (USA)

Prevalence of Proteinuria

At least two studies have looked at the prevalence of proteinuria in Mexican Americans as compared with non-Hispanic whites. After adjusting for age and duration of diabetes, clinical proteinuria, defined as ≥1+ on the Ames Albustix test, was 2.82 times more prevalent in Mexican American diabetic subjects as compared with non-Hispanic white diabetic subjects in San Antonio [95% confidence interval (CI) 1.05, 7.55; p = 0.039] and 1.58 times more prevalent as compared with non-Hispanic whites in Wisconsin (95% CI 1.05, 2.4; p = 0.017) [6]. The prevalence of microalbuminuria (>30 mg/l) was also significantly higher in Mexican American diabetic subjects (odds ratio 3.54, 95% CI = 1.28, 9.81; p = 0.015) [6]. In contrast, in the San Luis Valley in southern Colorado, no difference was found in the occurrence of nephropathy (elevated creatinine, proteinuria or microalbuminuria) between Mexican Americans and non-Hispanic whites [7].

Albuminuria Prior to Onset of NIDDM

In insulin-dependent diabetes mellitus, (IDDM), microalbuminuria is a marker for the onset of nephropathy. In NIDDM, a recent report from Finland [8] suggests that microalbuminuria may be part of the prediabetic or insulin-resistant state. Although no data are available among Mexican Americans, among Mexicans studied in the Mexico City Diabetes Study [9], higher prevalences of microalbuminuria were found in individuals with either a parental history of diabetes or impaired glucose tolerance. These data suggest that public health measures to prevent NIDDM nephropathy will have to address not only the diabetic but the prediabetic state as well.

Incidence of Diabetic End-Stage Renal Disease (ESRD)

In 1987 Ferguson et al. [10] reported that Hispanics in south-central Los Angeles, the majority of whom are Mexican American, did not have a higher crude incidence of ESRD than non-Hispanic whites during the years 1980–1983. However, this study was limited to a small geographic region and was not age adjusted. In 1993, Ferguson and Morrisey [11] reported that the crude incidence rates of ESRD became higher in Mexican Americans in 1984 and remained between African Americans and non-Hispanic whites through 1990. 37% of the Hispanic ESRD was from diabetes as compared with 19% among whites and 30% among blacks. The age at onset of diabetic ESRD was also lower for Hispanics (54 vs. 60 years for whites).

In 1988, using a statewide ESRD data base in Texas [12], we reported that the incidence of total ESRD was three times higher in Mexican Americans as compared with non-Hispanic whites in Texas and the incidence of diabetes-related ESRD six times higher. Age-specific indicence suggested that the excess in diabetes-related ESRD was from NIDDM, since the excess was found only in the older age groups, and the gap widened with increasing age [12]. Figure 1 displays age-specific incidence ratios for Mexican Americans and African Americans as compared with non-Hispanic whites.

For the years 1982–1989, the Colorado State Department of Health also reported an excess of diabetes-related ESRD among Hispanics [13]: 3.7 times using a general population denominator and 1.8 times using a diabetic denominator (i.e., adjusting for the higher prevalence of diabetes). Perhaps even more concerning was that the greatest increase in rates was found in Hispanics (770 as compared with 440% among blacks and 190%

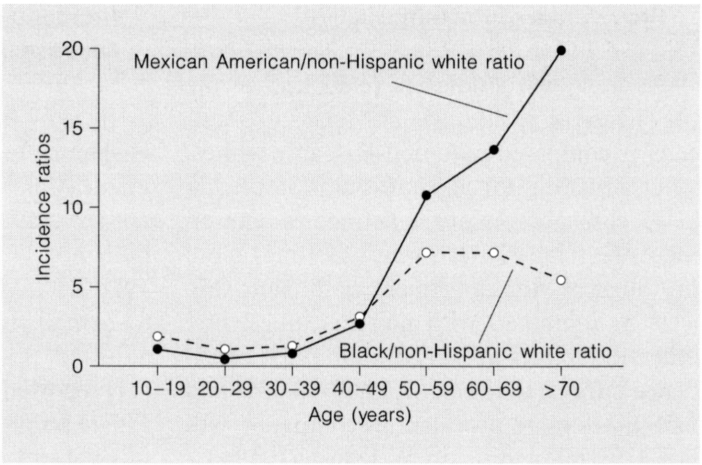

Fig. 1. Age-specific racial incidence ratios for diabetes-related ESRD in Texas, 1980–1982. [From ref. 12, with permission.]

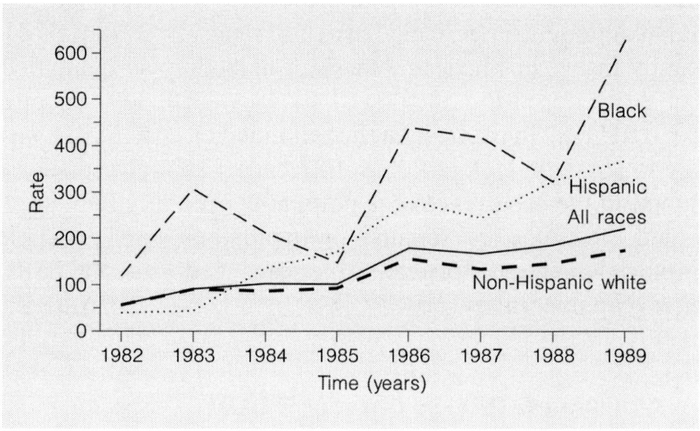

Fig. 2. Age-adjusted incidence rate (per 100,000 population with diabetes, adjusted to the 1980 US standard population with diabetes) of diabetes-related ESRD treatment by race and ethnicity – Colorado, 1982–1989. [From ref. 13, with permission.]

among non-Hispanic whites; fig. 2). While the US Renal Data System has not had a Hispanic marker until this year, their data reporting regional variation shows high rates (95th to 100th percentile) in southern California, Arizona, and the border regions of Texas, all areas with high concentrations of Mexican Americans [14].

Chiapella and Feldman [15] reported the incidence of ESRD using HCFA data for males with Hispanic surnames and found considerable regional variation in diagnoses. From 1985 to 1989, the percentage of ESRD due to diabetes was 50 for the Mexico border states, 36 for New York, 32 for Florida, and 41 for Puerto Rico [15]. These data indicate a variation among Hispanic subgroups in the risk of developing diabetic ESRD [15], not surprising given their variation in the prevalence of diabetes.

Incidence of IDDM and NIDDM ESRD

In the data bases reported above, IDDM and NIDDM could not be distinguished. To address this issue, we undertook a population-based study on the incidence of diabetes-relat-

Table 1. Age-adjusted annual incidence of treatment of diabetic ESRD (per 1,000,000 general population: San Antonio and Dallas, 1987–1991) [from ref. 16, with permission]

	Non-Hispanic whites	African Americans	Mexican Americans
Total diabetics			
Rate (95% CI)	53.6 (40.2–67.1)	350.9 (266.2–435.5)[b]	327.9 (263.2–392.6)[b]
Relative risk (95% CI)[a]		6.5 (4.6–9.3)	6.1 (4.4–8.4)
NIDDM			
Rate (95% CI)[a]	34.3 (23.4–45.3)	318.7 (236.7–400.6)[b]	316.8 (252.9–380.7)[b]
Relative risk (95% CI)[a]		9.3 (6.2–14.0)	9.2 (6.3–13.5)
IDDM			
Rate (95% CI)[a]	19.3 (11.5–27.1)	32.2 (11.0–53.4)	11.1 (0.9–21.3)
Relative risk (95% CI)[a]		1.7 (0.8–3.6)	0.6 (0.2–1.6)

[a] Comparison with non-Hispanic whites.
[b] $p < 0.00001$.

Table 2. Age-adjusted annual incidence of treatment of diabetic ESRD (per 100,000 diabetic population: San Antonio and Dallas, 1987–1991) [from ref. 16, with permission]

	Non-Hispanic whites	African Americans	Mexican Americans
Total DM diabetics			
Rate (95% CI)[a]	125.5 (83.8–167.2)	193.7 (141.2–246.2)[b]	117.8 (87.8–147.8)
Relative risk (95% CI)[a]		1.5 (1.0–2.4)	0.9 (0.6–1.4)
NIDDM			
rate (95% CI)[a]	41.5 (22.6–60.4)	155.7 (114.5–196.9)[d]	103.8 (77.3–130.4)[c]
Relative risk (95% CI)[a]		3.8 (2.2–6.4)	2.5 (1.5–4.2)
IDDM			
Rate (95% CI)[a]	84.0 (46.8–121.2)	38.0 (5.45–70.6)	14.0 (0–28.0)[c]
Relative risk (95% CI)[a]		0.45 (0.2–1.2)	0.2 (0.1–0.5)

[a] Comparison with non-Hispanic whites.
[b] $p < 0.05$; [c] $p < 0.001$; [d] $p < 0.0001$.

ed ESRD by diabetic type for three ethnic groups in Dallas and San Antonio, Texas [16]. The majority of diabetic ESRD in all ethnic/racial groups was from NIDDM [16]. The proportion represented by NIDDM is significantly higher for Mexican Americans (93%) and African Americans (84%) as compared with non-Hispanic whites (60%). The higher rate of diabetic ESRD was confirmed in the Mexican American as compared with the non-Hispanic white general population, and the excess risk was from NIDDM and not IDDM (tables 1, 2).

Risk Factors

Given the excess risk observed, the next question is why are Mexican Americans at increased risk of diabetic nephropathy. Mexican Americans have an earlier onset of their NIDDM than non-Hispanic whites which may decrease the competing mortality risks leaving a longer time to develop nephropathy [17]. The data by Ferguson et al. [10] and Ferguson and Morrisey [11] regarding the younger age at onset of ESRD lend credence to this hypothesis. Haffner et al. [17] found that Mexican Americans with diabetes, whether newly diagnosed or previously diagnosed, had higher glucose levels than non-Hispanic whites. Mexican Americans have not been found to have higher levels of hypertension, but for those who have hypertension, the control is worse [18]. Dietary protein intake was not found to be correlated with clinical proteinuria in Mexican Americans [19]. Lack of health insurance covering outpatient visits was found to correlate with proteinuria in Mexican Americans with diabetes [20]. No data have been published regarding familial clustering or genetic risks for nephropathy in Mexican Americans.

Haffner et al. [6] attempted to adjust for risk factors and see if there was any remaining excess risk for Mexican Americans. Using only previously diagnosed patients in the analysis, after controlling for duration of diabetes, insulin therapy, and prevalence of hypertension, the ethnic difference in proteinuria was still highly significant. Similar findings occurred with microalbuminuria, adjusting for age, duration of diabetes, systolic blood pressure, fasting glucose, and smoking [6].

Other risk factor data for the incidence of proteinuria in the San Luis Valley cohort and for ESRD from a case-control study in San Antonio and Dallas should be published soon.

Survival on Treatment for ESRD

Using data from the Texas Kidney Health Program, a statewide data base, Mexican Americans' survival on treatment for ESRD was compared with that of non-Hispanic whites. Among those with diabetic ESRD and after age adjustment, Mexican Americans were 23% less likely to die prematurely than non-Hispanic whites [21]. Table 3 presents age-adjusted data for all etiologies and treatment types by ethnic/racial group. In the multivariate model for all ESRD and types of treatment, Mexican Americans retained a highly significant advantage (hazard ratio = 0.47) in survival [21] (table 4). Survival data on a cohort of 638 diabetic ESRD patients in San Antonio and Dallas will soon be published. Preliminary data [22] reconfirmed that Mexican Americans with diabetic ESRD have a longer survival on hemodialysis, but that among those with NIDDM only, there were no ethnic differences in survival.

Conclusions

Mexican Americans have higher rates of diabetic ESRD than non-Hispanic whites. This excess is due to their increased prevalence of NIDDM and to known (poorer glycemic control, poorer hypertension control, lack of health insurance) as well as yet to be identified risk factors. Further, microalbuminuria may occur even prior to the development of frank diabetes, either as part of the insulin-resistant state or secondary to impaired glucose tolerance. In addition to having more ESRD, Mexican Americans have better survival on treatment for ESRD, leading to a large and growing public health burden. Prevention strategies must be forthcoming such as prevention of NIDDM itself, screening and early treatment of NIDDM,

Table 3. Hazard ratio for death compared to non-Hispanic whites stratified by disease type and treatment type (age adjusted) [from ref. 21, with permission]

	African American		Mexican American	
	hazard ratio	95% CI	hazard ratio	95% CI
Disease type				
All etiologies (n = 11,958)	0.71	0.67, 0.76	0.93	0.88, 0.99
Diabetes (n = 3,260)	0.55	0.48, 0.63	0.77	0.69, 0.86
Hypertension (n = 2,951)	0.65	0.58, 0.74	0.82	0.69, 0.96
Glomerulonephritis (n = 1,840)	0.86	0.70, 1.06	0.87	0.72, 1.05
Other (n = 3,907)	0.85	0.75, 0.95	0.90	0.80, 1.01
Treatment type				
Center hemodialysis (n = 9,848)	0.66	0.61, 0.70	0.89	0.84, 0.95
Home hemodialysis (n = 198)	1.11	0.53, 2.33	2.33	1.05, 5.15
Transplantation (n = 1,168)	0.98	0.65, 1.47	0.62	0.39, 1.00
Continuous ambulatory peritoneal dialysis (n = 730)	0.80	0.54, 1.19	0.81	0.56, 1.16

Table 4. Multivariate model for survival comparing all others to diabetic non-Hispanic whites (n = 11,556) [from ref. 21, with permission]

Predictor variable	Hazard ratio	p
Age (10-year interval)	1.30[a]	0.000
Mexican American	0.47	0.000
African American	0.90	0.501[b]
Disease other	0.57	0.000
Disease glomerulonephritis	0.53	0.000
Disease hypertension	0.66	0.000
Center size	0.93	0.010
Transplantation	0.37	0.000
Continuous ambulatory peritoneal dialysis	0.68	0.000
Mexican American age	1.07[a]	0.012
African American age	0.93[a]	0.000
Mexican American diseases other	1.19[a]	0.021
African American diseases other	1.35[a]	0.000

Required p = 0.10 to enter the model for the sample; sex showed no univariate association and was not included in the model.

[a] Calculated relative to each increasing age category.

[b] African Americans were kept in the model to preserve the structure of the variable race.

and screening and treatment of microalbuminuria. Lack of access to health care, in part due to lack of insurance coverage, may make such strategies hard to implement.

Acknowledgments

This work was funded by grants from the RGK Foundation, National Institutes of Health (R01 DK 38392), Agency for Health Care Policy and Research (U01 HS07397) and from the Texas Diabetes Council.

References

1 Stern MP, Rosenthal M, Haffner SM, et al: Sex difference in the effects of sociocultural status on diabetes and cardiovascular risk factors in Mexican Americans. Am J Epidemiol 1984;120:834–851.

2 Joos SK, Mueller WH, Hanis CL, et al: Diabetes alert study: Weight history and upper body obesity in diabetic and non-diabetic Mexican American adults. Ann Hum Biol 1984;11:167–171.

3 Marshall JA, Hamman RF, Baxter J, Mayer EJ, Fulton DL, Orleans M, Rewers M, Jones RH: Ethnic differences in risk factors associated with the prevalence of non-insulin-dependent diabetes mellitus: The San Luis Valley Diabetes Study. Am J Epidemiol 1993;137:706–718.

4 Haffner SM, Hazuda HP, Mitchell BD, Patterson JK, Stern MP: Increased incidence of type II diabetes mellitus in Mexican Americans. Diabetes Care 1991;14:102–108.

5 Baxter J, Hamman RF, López TK, Marshall JA, Hoag S, Swenson CJ: Excess incidence of known non-insulin-dependent diabetes mellitus (NIDDM) in Hispanics compared with non-Hispanic whites in the San Luis Valley, Colorado. Ethn Dis 1993;3:11–21.

6 Haffner SM, Mitchell BD, Pugh JA, Stern MP, Kozlowski MK, Hazuda HP, Patterson JK, Klein R: Proteinuria in Mexican American and non-Hispanic whites with NIDDM. Diabetes Care 1989;12:530–536.

7 Hamman RF, Franklin GA, Mayer EJ, Marshall SM, Marshall JA, Baxter J, Kahn LB: Microvascular complications of NIDDM in Hispanics and non-Hispanic whites: The San Luis Valley Diabetes Study. Diabetes Care 1991;14:655–664.

8 Mykkanen L, Haffner SM, Kuusisto J, Pyorala K, Lakso M: Microalbuminuria precedes the development of NIDDM. Diabetes 1994;43:552–557.

9 Haffner SM, Gonzales C, Valdez RA, Mykkanen L, Hazuda HP, Mitchell BD, Monterrosa A, Stern MP: Is microalbuminuria part of the prediabetic state? The Mexico City Diabetes Study. Diabetologia 1993; 36:1002–1006.

10 Ferguson R, Grim CE, Opgenorth TJ: The epidemiology of end-stage renal disease: The six-year south-central Los Angeles experience. Am J Public Health 1987;7:864–865.

11 Ferguson R, Morrisey E: Risk factors for end-stage renal disease among minorities. Transplant Proc 1993;25:2415–2420.

12 Pugh JA, Stern MP, Haffner SM, Eifler CW, Zapata M: Excess incidence of treatment of end-stage renal disease in Mexican Americans. Am J Epidemiol 1988;127:135–144.

13 Hamman RF, Turak A, Stiles SK, Finucane FF, Michael SL, Garrett CJ, Meng C, Gabella BA: Incidence of treatment for end-stage renal disease attributed to diabetes mellitus, by race/ethnicity – Colorado, 1982–1989. MMWR Morb Mortal Wkly Rep 1992;6:41:845–848.

14 Foxman B, Moulton LH, Wolfe RA, Guire KE, Port FK, Hawthorne VM: Geographic variation in the incidence of related end-stage renal disease. J Am Soc Nephrol 1991;2: 1144–1152.

15 Chiapella AP, Feldman HI: End-stage renal disease in Hispanic males. Am J Public Health 1995;85: 1001–1004.

16 Pugh JA, Medina RA, Cornell JC, Basu S: Non-insulin-dependent diabetes is the major cause of diabetic end-stage renal disease: More evidence from a tri-ethnic community. Diabetes 1995;44:1375–1380.

17 Haffner SM, Rosenthal M, Hazuda HP, et al: Evaluation of three potential screening tests for diabetes mellitus in a bi-ethnic population. Diabetes Care 1984;7:347–353.

18 Haffner SM, Morales PA, Hazuda HP, Stern MP: Level of control of hypertension in Mexican Americans and non-Hispanic whites. Hypertension 1993;21:83–88.

19 Jameel N, Pugh JA: Dietary protein intake and proteinuria among type II diabetics in a population-based study. Diabetes Care 1992;15: 178–183.

20 Pugh JA, Tuley M, Hazuda HP, Stern MP: The influence of outpatient insurance coverage on the microvascular complications of non-insulin-dependent diabetes in Mexican Americans. J Diabetes Complications 1992;6:236–241.

21 Pugh JA, Tuley MR, Basu S: Survival among Mexican-Americans, non-Hispanic whites, and African Americans with end-stage renal disease: The emergence of a minority pattern of increased incidence and prolonged survival. Am J Kidney Dis 1994;23:803–807.

22 Medina RA, Pugh JA, Cornell JC: Predictors of survival in patients with type II diabetes-related end-stage renal disease (abstract). J Gen Intern Med 1995;10(suppl 4):47.

Blood Purification

Blood Purif 1996;14:293–304

Access of Native Americans to Renal Transplantation in Arizona and New Mexico

Andrew Narva[a]
Sharon Stiles[b]
Shelley Karp[b]
Alice Turak[b]

[a] Indian Health Service, Albuquerque, N. Mex.;
[b] Intermountain End-Stage Renal Disease Network No. 15, Denver, Colo., USA

Key Words

Arizona, renal transplantation
End-stage renal disease
Native Americans
New Mexico, renal transplantation

Abstract

Lower rates of transplantation among minority groups are a nationally recognized phenomenon. Native Americans (NA) nationally have nearly four times the risk of end-stage renal disease (ESRD) as compared with white (W) Americans and are significantly overrepresented in the Network 15 ESRD population. To understand more about NA and W transplant rates, we looked at all reported Arizona (AZ) and New Mexico (NM) resident cases from the Network No. 15 data base. Age of onset, sex, primary diagnosis, payment source, transplant donor source, and other factors were examined. NA experienced a slightly earlier onset of ESRD than W, and diabetes mellitus was the primary ESRD diagnosis for 63–73% of NA and for 34–39% of W. Because age distribution and frequency of diabetes mellitus of the NA ESRD population differ from those of W in the Network, age-specific and diagnosis-specific transplant rates were examined. Age-adjusted transplant rates per 100 ESRD patients for AZ were 16.4 (NA) and 21.0 (W) and for NM 14.2 (NA) and 22.4 (W). Diagnosis-specific age-adjusted transplant rates for patients with the primary diagnoses of diabetes mellitus and glomerulonephritis, the two most common causes of ESRD among NA, showed a large difference between W and NA rates. Age-adjusted rates for diabetics were: AZ 8.5% (NA) and 14.5% (W); NM 9.8% (NA) and 15.9% (W). Age-adjusted rates for patients with glomerulonephritis were: AZ 23.7% (NA) and 28.0% (W); NM 22.3% (NA) and 33.0% (W). In all comparisons and in both the W and NA ESRD populations, women were transplanted at lower rates than men. NA experienced a greater delay from onset of treated ESRD to transplant than W. Payment source and transplant donor source did not appear to be significantly different between NA and W. The lower transplant rates in NA versus W in Network No. 15 cannot be explained by age- or diagnosis-specific factors.

This work was developed under Health Care Financing Administration Contract No. 500-91-0020.

KARGER

E-Mail karger@karger.ch
Fax + 41 61 306 12 34
http://www.karger.ch

0253–5068/96/0144–0293$10.00/0

Andrew S. Narva, MD
IHS Kidney Disease Program
801 Vassar Drive, NE
Albuquerque, NM 87106 (USA)

Table 1. ESRD Network No. 15: Native Americans as percent of total population and treated ESRD patients by state as of December 31, 1990

	State						Network No. 15
	Arizona	Colorado	Nevada	New Mexico	Utah	Wyoming	
% of total population in state who are Native American	5.6	0.8	1.6	8.9	1.4	2.1	3.5
Total patients on dialysis	1,956	1,125	430	736	380	87	4,817
% of dialysis patients who are Native American	19.8	1.9	4.0	29.6	5.3	6.9	14.2
Total patients with transplant	542	510	67	231	398	60	2,096
% of transplant patients who are Native American	11.1	0.6	3.0	17.0	1.8	1.7	5.7

End-stage renal disease (ESRD) treatment rates, both crude and adjusted for age, race, and sex, increased steadily through the 1980s in the United States. The increase has been more dramatic in Native Americans than in whites. The United States Renal Data System (USRDS) reports that between 1982 and 1989, the age- and sex-adjusted incidence rates of reported ESRD therapy increased 66% for whites and 150% for Native Americans. At the same time, these adjusted rates for Native Americans increased from 2.5 times that for whites in 1982 to 3.9 times that of whites in 1989 [1]. (Data reported by the USRDS are from the Health Care Financing Administration ESRD Medical Information System which includes approximately 92% of the ESRD patients who are on Medicare).

Native American ESRD patients, like other minorities, are less likely to have a functioning transplant than whites [2]. About half of all Native Americans with treated ESRD live in the six states comprising ESRD Network No. 15, making the Network an ideal place to examine some reasons for the lower transplant rate among Native American treated ESRD patients. Treatment providers report tribal identification to the Network for Native American patients, increasing the specificity of the data and mitigating against ethnic misclassification, a common problem with data on Native Americans with ESRD. The accuracy of the data in the Network is constantly being improved as better information is reported by treatment providers. Because of the relative abundance and the quality of Native American data in the Network, the remainder of the discussion focuses on data collected and maintained by Network No. 15.

Patients and Methods

Native Americans are overrepresented in the ESRD population as compared with their proportions in the general population of each state [3]. This overrepresentation is more pronounced in dialysis patients than in transplant patients. In the six states comprising the Network, 3.5% of the population is Native American; in the ESRD Network, 14.2% of the dialysis

Table 2. ESRD Network No. 15: ESRD treatment by state of residence of living Native American and white patients as of December 31, 1990

	State						Network No. 15
	Arizona	Colorado	Nevada	New Mexico	Utah	Wyoming	
Native American	446	24	19	256	27	7	799
Dialysis	386	21	17	217	20	6	680
Transplant	60	3	2	39	7	1	119
% transplant	13.5	12.5	10.5	15.2	25.9	14.3	14.9
White	1,405	1,120	312	328	686	121	4,274
Dialysis	1,033	736	262	229	324	67	2,723
Transplant	372	384	50	99	362	54	1,551
% transplant	26.5	34.3	16.0	30.2	52.8	44.6	36.3

patients and 5.7% of the transplant patients are Native Americans (table 1). Validation studies have indicated that underidentification of Native Americans in disease registries is likely, so that the Native American incidence may actually be higher than reported [4].

The crude renal transplant rate for Native Americans in the Network and in each of the six states is consistently lower than for whites [3]. Table 2 shows, for each state and the Network, the number of living Native American and white patients who were on dialysis and transplanted as of December 31, 1990, and the transplant rate, computed as:

$$\frac{\text{number with transplant 12/31/90}}{\text{number on dialysis + number with transplant 12/31/90}}$$

Excluded from these calculations are persons who had a functioning transplant graft since before 1982; they have never been reported to the Network.

The crude transplant rate for whites is double that for Native Americans in both Arizona and New Mexico, the states with the greatest number of Native Americans. Networkwide, the transplant rate for whites is 2.4 times higher than for Native Americans. Utah and Wyoming both have very high transplant rates for whites as compared with the other states included in the Network (53 and 45%, respectively), accounting for the overall higher transplant rates for whites. These two states had higher proportions of patients receiving their first transplants from living-related donors than the other states in the Network, possibly contributing to their high transplant rates. Because of the very small number of Native Americans in four states in the Network, only data from New Mexico and Arizona will be further discussed.

In an effort to understand more about Native American and white patients in ESRD Network No. 15, we looked at *all* reported Arizona and New Mexico resident cases from the Network No. 15 data base (whether currently living or dead). We examined several data items, such as age at onset of treated ESRD, primary diagnosis, source of payment for medical care, and donor source, to try to find differences between Native American and white ESRD patients that might explain the higher transplant rates among whites.

Results

Age at Onset of Treated ESRD

Data in table 3 indicate that there are differences in age of onset of treated ESRD in Arizona and New Mexico. In Arizona, the percentage of white patients under age 45 years at onset of treated ESRD is slightly higher than the percentage of Native American patients. Over the next couple of decades of age, the Native American treated ESRD pop-

Table 3. ESRD Network No. 15: age at onset of treated ESRD in Native American and white patients (% of all reported cases)

Age at onset, years	Arizona		New Mexico	
	Native American	white	Native American	white
Total persons	1,039	5,448	553	1,811
<5	0.1	0.3	0.0	0.3
5–9	0.2	0.4	0.2	0.3
10–14	0.9	0.7	0.5	1.4
15–19	0.8	1.3	1.8	2.0
20–24	1.5	2.8	2.0	2.9
25–29	1.8	3.8	1.4	4.1
30–34	3.2	4.1	3.3	5.1
35–39	4.3	4.8	5.8	5.3
40–44	5.7	5.0	8.5	6.4
45–49	12.2	5.4	8.7	7.1
50–54	14.2	7.1	12.3	8.3
55–59	15.6	9.9	15.6	10.0
60–64	11.5	13.2	13.4	12.3
65–69	11.8	13.7	10.7	12.9
70–74	8.1	12.7	8.1	11.5
75–79	5.1	8.8	4.0	6.8
80 and over	2.2	5.5	3.3	2.8
Unknown	0.8	0.6	0.5	0.6

ulation grows dramatically. About 30% of both the Native American and white patients are under 50 years of age. Forty-five percent of the Native Americans and 36% of the whites are under age 55; 61% of the Native Americans and 46% of the whites are under 65. These findings coincide with the earlier onset of ESRD reported elsewhere for Native Americans compared with US whites [5]. A similar pattern holds for New Mexico patients, with the age discrepancy beginning slightly later, and the differences being slightly less striking.

Primary ESRD Diagnosis

Table 4 displays the primary diagnosis of patients in the Network data base. 63–76% of the Native Americans and 34–40% of the whites are reported to have diabetic nephropathy. Diabetic nephropathy is more common in Arizona than in New Mexico Native American ESRD patients. Females, both Native American and white, contribute more heavily to this diagnostic group than do males.

The primary ESRD diagnosis may not be accurate in every case. It is possible that many of the Native Americans with reported primary hypertension or unknown diagnosis may actually have glomerulonephritis. In addition, Native Americans who are reported to have diabetes may have that disease in addition to glomerulonephritis as a comorbid condition. Not infrequently, Native American patients present with diabetes, chronic renal failure, and bilaterally small kidneys not appropriate for biopsy. Distinguishing diabetes as a primary etiology from a comorbid state can be difficult in this situation.

Table 4. ESRD Network No. 15: primary diagnosis in Native American and white patients by sex (%; all reported cases)

Primary diagnosis	Arizona		New Mexico	
	Native American	white	Native American	white
All cases				
Total persons	1,039	5,448	553	1,811
Hypertension	5.6	20.4	6.9	17.8
Glomerulonephritis	10.3	19.7	15.2	19.8
Diabetic nephropathy	72.2	34.4	62.6	39.0
Other	5.7	19.7	7.2	16.3
Unknown	6.3	5.8	8.1	7.1
Males				
Total persons	475	3,084	241	986
Hypertension	6.5	22.2	7.1	19.8
Glomerulonephritis	12.4	22.2	16.2	20.8
Diabetic nephropathy	65.9	30.5	59.8	36.0
Other	7.8	19.2	9.1	16.1
Unknown	7.4	5.9	7.9	7.3
Females				
Total persons	564	2,362	311	825
Hypertension	4.8	18.0	6.8	15.5
Glomerulonephritis	8.5	16.4	14.5	18.5
Diabetic nephropathy	77.5	39.6	64.6	42.7
Other	3.9	20.2	5.8	16.5
Unknown	5.3	5.8	8.4	6.8

Sex unknown for 2 Arizona white patients and 1 New Mexico Native American patient.

Medical Coverage for Treated ESRD Patients

The payment source in the data base is the most current primary payer for each patient. In the Network data base, more than 75% of Native American and over 83% of white patients are on Medicare (table 5). An additional 4–6% are Medicare eligible. Care for only 4% of Arizona Native American and for only 2% of New Mexico Native American ESRD patients is paid by the Indian Health Service. Fewer than 1% of the ESRD patients are reported to have no payment source.

Transplant Rates

Table 6 shows that in the Network data base for all cases, the transplant rate for whites is higher than that for Native Americans: in Arizona by more than 35% and in New Mexico by over 75%. In Arizona the discrepancy is almost entirely found in women. In New Mexico the inconsistency is apparent for both males and females, but the difference is greater for women. Table 6 also reveals that women seem to be transplanted at a lower rate than men, especially among the Native American patients. Lower transplant rates for wom-

Table 5. ESRD Network No. 15: primary payment source of Native American and white patients by sex (%; all reported cases)

Primary payment source	Arizona		New Mexico	
	Native American	white	Native American	white
All cases				
Total persons	1,039	5,448	553	1,811
Medicare eligible	6.4	5.1	6.5	4.2
Medicare	76.2	83.9	77.2	86.3
Indian Health Service	4.1	0.0	1.8	0.0
Other/unknown	13.3	11.0	14.5	9.5
Males				
Total persons	475	3,084	241	986
Medicare eligible	6.5	4.7	5.4	4.5
Medicare	81.7	83.1	76.8	84.2
Indian Health Service	2.7	0.0	2.5	0.0
Other/unknown	9.1	12.2	15.3	11.3
Females				
Total persons	564	2,362	311	825
Medicare eligible	6.2	5.6	7.4	3.9
Medicare	71.6	84.9	77.5	88.7
Indian Health Service	5.3	0.0	1.3	0.0
Other/unknown	16.9	9.5	13.8	7.4

Primary payment source is most current data obtained by Network No. 15. Sex unknown for 2 Arizona white patients and 1 New Mexico Native American patient.

en than for men were also foundby other researchers and should be further investigated [6, 7].

Age-Specific and Age-Adjusted Transplant Rates

Because the age distribution of the Native American ESRD population differs from that of whites in the Network, transplant rates used for comparison should be age specific or age adjusted rather than crude. Table 7 presents crude, age-specific, and age-adjusted rates for all cases. Differences in transplant rates that are due to dissimilar age distributions will disappear when a comparison is made of age-specific rates. The cases were divided into five age groups: <20, 21–44, 45–64, 65–74, and 75 years and over. The age-specific rates (number of transplants/number of patients in an age-group) for Native Americans and whites are different in both Arizona and New Mexico. Age adjusting the rates allows for comparison of one rate for each patient group. The age-specific rates are applied to a 'standard' population, so differences in age distributions are not an issue. For the 'standard' population, we used the 1990 Network prevalent population. Consistently,

Table 6. ESRD Network No. 15: patients ever transplanted among Native American and white patients by sex (all reported cases)

Patients ever transplanted	Arizona		New Mexico	
	Native American	white	Native American	white
All cases				
Total persons	1,039	5,448	553	1,811
%	11.1	15.3	10.8	19.1
Males				
Total persons	475	3,084	241	986
%	15.8	16.7	13.7	20.9
Females				
Total persons	564	2,362	311	825
%	7.1	13.5	8.7	17.0

Sex unknown for 2 Arizona white patients and 1 New Mexico Native American patient.

Table 7. ESRD Network No. 15: crude, age-specific, and age-adjusted transplant rates per 100 ESRD patients (preliminary data)

Age at onset of treated ESRD years	Arizona		New Mexico	
	Native American	white	Native American	white
Total number of patients				
Total persons	1,031	5,417	550	1,800
<20	20	148	14	72
20–44	172	1,116	116	430
45–64	556	1,938	276	683
65–74	207	1,438	104	441
75 and over	76	777		174
Crude transplant rate				
Total	11.1	15.3	10.8	19.1
Age-specific transplant rate				
<20	60.0	64.9	50.0	63.9
20–44	34.9	44.2	31.0	43.7
45–64	6.8	11.1	6.2	15.1
65–74	1.9	1.2	0.0	1.6
75 and over	0.0	0.0	0.0	0.6
Age-adjusted transplant rate				
Total	16.4	21.0	14.2	22.4

Age-adjusted by the direct method to the ESRD Network No. 15 'standard million' 12/31/90 prevalent population. Excludes 8 Arizona Native American, 31 Arizona white, 3 New Mexico Native American, and 11 New Mexico white patients with age at onset of ESRD unknown.

Table 8. ESRD Network No. 15: primary diagnosis – patients ever transplanted (%; all reported cases)

Primary diagnosis – transplanted patients	Arizona		New Mexico	
	Native American	white	Native American	white
All cases				
Total persons	115	834	60	346
Hypertension	8.7	11.0	8.3	9.0
Glomerulonephritis	32.2	33.3	38.3	38.2
Diabetic nephropathy	35.7	22.7	33.3	24.6
Other	9.6	26.3	10.0	22.5
Unknown	13.9	6.7	10.0	5.8
Males				
Total persons	75	514	33	206
Hypertension	9.3	12.1	6.1	10.2
Glomerulonephritis	32.0	36.0	36.4	38.3
Diabetic nephropathy	33.3	22.6	39.4	26.2
Other	12.0	23.2	9.1	18.4
Unknown	13.3	6.2	9.1	6.8
Females				
Total persons	40	320	27	140
Hypertension	7.5	9.4	11.1	7.1
Glomerulonephritis	32.5	29.1	40.7	37.9
Diabetic nephropathy	40.0	22.8	25.9	22.1
Other	5.0	31.3	11.1	28.6
Unknown	15.0	7.5	11.1	4.3

the age-adjusted transplant rate for white patients was higher than the age-adjusted rate for Native American patients.

Diagnosis of Transplanted Patients

Because patients with some primary ESRD diagnoses are better candidates than others for transplantation, we looked at transplanted patients to see what differences there are in their diagnoses. In table 8, patients with diabetic nephropathy are underrepresented in the transplanted patients and those with glomerulonephritis overrepresented, more so in Native Americans than in whites.

Age-Specific and Age-Adjusted Transplant Rates by Diagnosis

Because transplant rates would be expected to be dissimilar in different diagnostic groups, as shown in table 8, we computed age-specific and age-adjusted transplant rates for the two large diagnostic groups: glomerulonephritis (table 9) and diabetic nephropath (table 10). Table 9 shows that in Arizona the age-specific transplant rate for 20- to 44-year-old Native American and white patients with glomerulonephritis was about the same: 53–54%. The age-adjusted rates remained higher in whites than in Native Americans. In Ari-

Table 9. ESRD Network No. 15: crude, age-specific, and age-adjusted transplant rates per 100 ESRD patients with glomerulonephritis (all reported cases; preliminary data)

Age at onset of treated ESRD	Arizona		New Mexico	
	Native American	white	Native American	white
Total number of patients				
Total persons	104	1,066	84	353
<20	10	65	5	29
20–44	55	296	40	116
45–64	24	339	25	131
65–75	11	242	8	61
75 and over	4	124	6	16
Crude transplant rate				
Total	34.6	25.9	27.4	36.9
Age-specific transplant rate				
<20	50.0	60.0	60.0	82.8
20–44	52.7	54.4	35.0	61.2
45–64	12.5	20.6	24.0	27.5
65–74	0.0	2.5	0.0	0.0
75 and over	0.0	0.0	0.0	0.0
Age-adjusted transplant rate				
Total	23.7	28.0	22.3	33.0

Age-adjusted by the direct method to the ESRD Network No. 15 'standard million' 12/31/90 prevalent population. Excludes 3 Arizona Native American, 7 Arizona white, and 5 New Mexico white patients with age at onset of ESRD unknown.

zona, the crude transplant rate for these patients was actually 37% higher in Native Americans than in whites, but age adjusting resulted in a 15% lower transplant rate for Native Americans. Among patients with diabetic nephropathy, age-adjusted transplant rates for white patients were typically twice that of Native American patients. Comorbid conditions may play a role.

Donor Source

Table 11 presents data on the source of the latest transplant for each patient. (The donor source for patients who had only one transplant is essentially the same as shown in this table). The distribution of sources for Native Americans and whites in the Network data base is virtually identical: 73-76% are cadaveric kidneys, and 17–23% are from living-related donors.

Delay from Onset of Treated ESRD to Transplant

Table 12 presents the time between onset of treated ESRD and transplant. Not only are Native Americans not transplanted as at high a rate as whites, they are also transplanted later after onset of treatment. Table 12 shows

Table 10. ESRD Network No. 15: crude, age-specific, and age-adjusted transplant rates per 100 ESRD patients with diabetic nephropathy (all reported cases; preliminary data)

Age at onset of treated ESRD	Arizona		New Mexico	
	Native American	white	Native American	white
Total number of patients				
Total persons	748	1,870	344	705
<20	1	3	0	5
20–44	79	418	41	161
45–64	459	817	207	325
65–74	159	479	75	177
75 and over	50	153	21	37
Crude transplant rate				
Total	5.5	10.1	5.8	12.0
Age-specific transplant rate				
<20	0.0	33.3	0.0	40.0
20–44	19.0	35.4	24.4	34.8
45–64	5.0	4.3	4.8	8.0
65–74	1.9	0.4	0.0	0.6
75 and over	0.0	0.0	0.0	0.0
Age-adjusted transplant rate				
Total	8.5	14.5	9.8	15.9

Age-adjusted by the direct method to the ESRD Network No. 15 'standard million' 12/31/90 prevalent population. Excludes 2 Arizona Native American, 6 Arizona white, 2 New Mexico Native American, and 2 New Mexico white patients with age at onset of ESRD unknown.

that Native Americans in both Arizona and New Mexico follow the same pattern; New Mexico white patients get their transplants slightly before Arizona patients. The difference in delay time for Native Americans versus whites in Arizona is about 4 months and is resolved by about 2 years and 6 months after onset of treatment. The difference in New Mexico is about 4–6 months, and Native Americans catch up to whites at about 3 years and 6 months to 4 years after onset of treatment.

Discussion

There are differences in transplant rates between Native American and white treated ESRD patients, both nationally and in Network No. 15. The Network collects data on about half the Native American treated patients in the nation. We looked at data for Arizona and New Mexico, the two states in the Network with most of the Native American population and treated ESRD patients. There were differences in age at onset of treated disease, primary diagnosis, and delay from onset to transplant. There were differences in trans-

Table 11. ESRD Network No. 15: donor source for latest transplant (%; all reported cases)

Latest donor source	Arizona		New Mexico	
	Native American	white	Native American	white
All cases				
Total persons	115	834	60	346
Cadaveric	75.7	72.9	73.3	74.9
Living related	19.1	20.6	23.3	16.8
Unrelated living	0.0	0.0	0.0	0.0
Unknown	05.2	6.5	3.3	8.4
Males				
Total persons	75	514	33	206
Cadaveric	70.7	74.5	84.8	76.2
Living related	22.7	18.1	15.2	16.5
Unrelated living	0.0	0.0	0.0	0.0
Unknown	6.7	7.4	0.0	7.3
Females				
Total persons	40	320	27	140
Cadaveric	85.0	70.3	59.3	72.9
Living related	12.5	24.7	33.3	17.1
Unrelated living	0.0	0.0	0.0	0.0
Unknown	2.5	5.0	7.4	10.0

plant rates, even when we triedto correct for primary diagnosis and age distributions. Further, there were differences in transplant rates between males and females of the same race and between races of the same sex.

The issue of lower transplant rates in Native Americans should be examined further. Other data that might be enlightening would include comorbid conditions, survival rates, and additional barriers to transplantation besides economic ones: cultural differences, difficulty with language, and provider attitudes, for example. Information regarding length of time patients spend on transplant waiting lists and crossmatch difficulty by race would be of interest, as well.

If further analyses fail to reveal that lower transplant rates for Native Americans are justified for medical reasons, interventions may be undertaken by Indian Health Service and/or ESRD Network No. 15 to attempt to increase access to transplantation for Native Americans.

Table 12. ESRD Network No. 15: time from onset of treated ESRD to first transplant of patients ever transplanted (% cumulated; all reported cases; preliminary data)

Time from onset of treated ESRD to transplant, months	Arizona		New Mexico	
	Native American	white	Native American	white
Total persons	95	665	56	263
<1	2.1	7.2	5.4	8.7
1	3.2	9.9	7.1	11.0
2	4.2	13.4	7.1	13.3
3	5.3	16.1	8.9	16.0
4	7.4	19.5	8.9	19.4
5	7.4	23.2	10.7	23.2
6	11.6	25.9	16.1	29.3
7	16.8	29.5	19.6	35.0
8	21.1	33.4	21.4	38.8
9	24.2	36.4	21.4	42.6
10	25.3	40.0	25.0	45.6
11	30.5	43.6	30.4	49.8
12	33.7	46.9	32.1	53.6
13–15	42.1	54.6	42.9	61.2
16–18	48.4	60.3	50.0	65.0
19–21	53.7	67.2	55.4	70.0
22–24	64.2	71.3	58.9	74.1
25–30	77.9	78.9	75.0	81.4
31–36	82.1	82.3	80.4	84.4
37–48	90.5	88.3	87.5	89.4
49–60	93.7	91.7	94.6	93.5
>60	100.0	100.0	100.0	100.0

Includes only patients with one transplant. Excludes 6 Arizona Native American, 52 Arizona white, 1 New Mexico Native American, and 25 New Mexico white patients without information.

References

1 United States Renal Data System: Annual Data Report. US Department of Health and Human Services, Public Health Service, National Institutes of Health, p A5.

2 United States Renal Data System: 1991 Annual Data Report. US Department of Health and Human Services, Public Health Service, National Institutes of Health, pp C1, C6, C7.

3 Selected Demographics – 1990. Intermountain End-Stage Renal Disease Network No. 15, Inc.

4 Newman JM, Marfin AA, Eggers PW, Helgerson SD: End-stage renal disease among Native Americans, 1983–86. Am J Public Health 1990; 80:318–319.

5 Hoy WE, Megill DM, Hughson MD: Epidemic renal disease of unknown etiology in the Zuni Indians. Am J Kidney Dis 1987;9:485–496.

6 Kjellstrand CM: Age, sex, and race inequality in renal transplantation. Arch Intern Med 1988;148:1305–1309.

7 Soucie JM, Neylan JF, McClellan W: Race and sex differences in the identification of candidates for renal transplantation. Am J Kidney Dis 1992;19:414–419.

Blood Purification

Blood Purif 1996;14:305–314

Stephen C. Textor

Division of Hypertension, Mayo Clinic, Rochester, Minn., USA

Atherosclerotic Renovascular Disease as a Cause of End-Stage Renal Disease: Cost Considerations

Key Words
Renal artery stenosis
Hypertension
Ischemic nephropathy
End-stage renal disease
Atherosclerosis
Renovascular disease

Abstract
Atherosclerotic vascular disease affects an increasing number of patients with end-stage renal disease. A review of comorbid atherosclerotic disease in 7,200 end-stage renal disease patients indicated that occlusive disease of the renal arteries may contribute to progressive renal failure in 1.34% of the US dialysis population or in 14% of the Caucasian patients with hypertensive nephrosclerosis. The costs of dialytic care in such patients exceed USD 87 million annually. The risks and costs of surgical revascularization of such patients are large, however. These data argue that prospective trials of intervention in atherosclerotic renal artery disease are urgently needed.

The potential for atherosclerotic renovascular disease to cause progressive renal failure presents a vexing challenge for nephrologists. No specific entry term appears for occlusive disease of the main renal artery in the diagnostic registry for the US, Renal Data Systems (USRDS) [1]. Yet, as the population reaching end-stage renal disease (ESRD) expands and ages, more patients than ever before have evident atherosclerotic disease extending to lower aorta and kidneys, potentially harboring critical vascular lesions.

Accumulating clinical experience indicates that renal artery revascularization can delay or prevent ESRD in some patients. An example of such a patient is shown in figure 1.

Rarely, revascularization in patients with ESRD already on dialysis has led to recovery of sufficient function to discontinue dialytic support [2, 3]. For this reason, ‘ischemic nephropathy’ is receiving increased attention as a potentially reversible cause of renal failure.

Prospective identification of patients losing renal function directly as a result of occult arterial disease affecting the kidneys is diffi-

KARGER

E-Mail karger@karger.ch
Fax + 41 61 306 12 34
http://www.karger.ch

Stephen C. Textor, MD
Division of Hypertension, W9A
Mayo Clinic
Rochester, MN 55905 (USA)

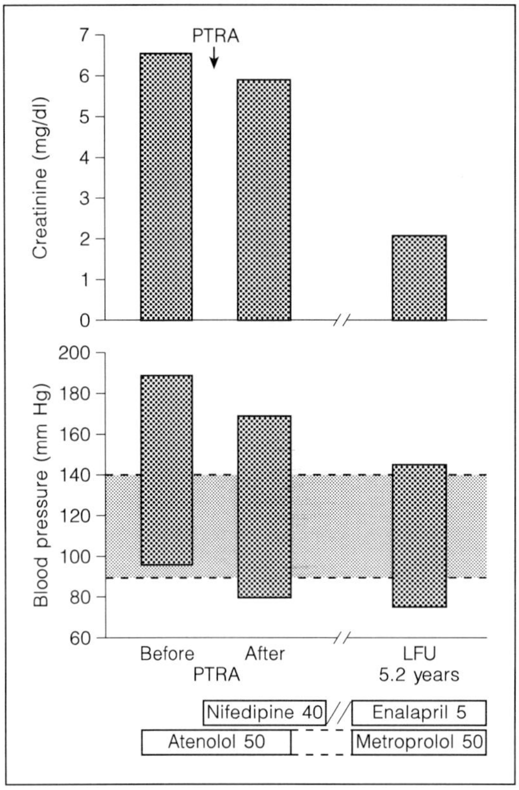

Fig. 1. Serum creatinine level before and after percutaneous transluminal renal angioplasty (PTRA) in a patient with bilateral atherosclerotic renal artery stenosis. The fall in creatinine from 6.3 to 1.7 mg/dl represented a clinical improvement in renal function which was sustained for more than 5 years and allowed improved blood pressure control. Angiotensin-converting enzyme inhibitors were administered during this period without adverse effects. LFU = Last follow-up (5.2 years after PTRA).

cult. The situation is made more complex by the fact that the hazards and costs of invasive studies and renal revascularization are substantial.

How many patients reaching ESRD in the US have critical occlusive disease of the renal arteries? Few data address this issue directly. Furthermore, it is not clear which patients might benefit from renal revascularization. Little is known regarding the costs and risks of intervention in such individuals.

The objective of the present paper is to examine several issues regarding the potential incidence and pathophysiology of ischemic renal disease, particularly as it applies to patients reaching ESRD. Data from the USRDS have been utilized to examine the frequency of comorbid vascular conditions in order to estimate the frequency of this disorder. These estimates may clarify relative cost considerations as they apply to managing such patients.

Definition and Incidence

Atherosclerosis commonly involves the descending aorta. Postmortem studies and review of aortograms obtained for other reasons indicate that some degree of renal artery stenosis is present in 45–65% of the patients over age 60 [4, 5], particularly if hypertension or azotemia (reflected by a creatinine level ≥1.5 mg/dl) are present.

It must be emphasized that stenotic vascular lesions have little, if any, hemodynamic effects until the luminal diameter is reduced to 75–80% [6]. For this reason, the term 'critical' arterial stenosis has been applied to lesions of sufficient degree to reduce blood flow or to reduce flow and poststenotic perfusion pressure during reductions in systemic arterial pressure. Studies using provocative maneuvers, such as blood pressure reduction during nitroprusside infusion (fig. 2), can identify functional limitations posed by vascular lesions to the kidney [7, 8].

These studies establish further that revascularization of the kidney in some instances can relieve critical dependence upon arterial pressure. However, such studies are difficult to perform and are limited to patients with measurable renal function.

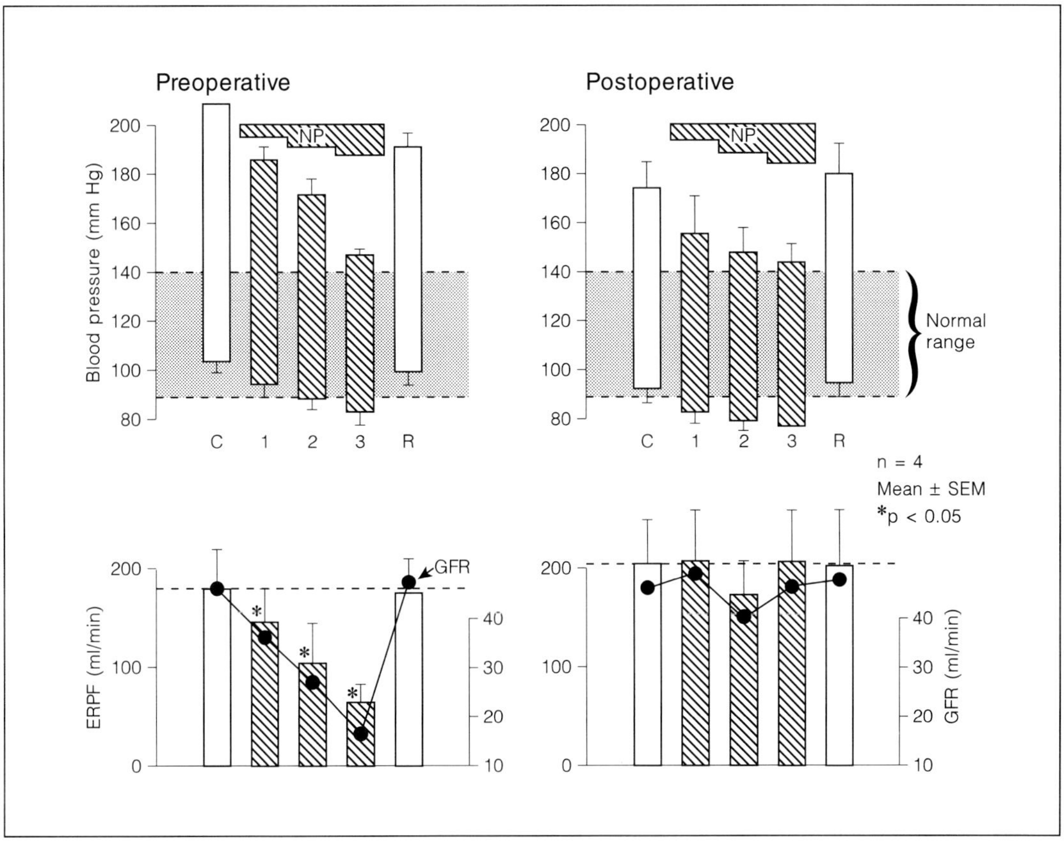

a

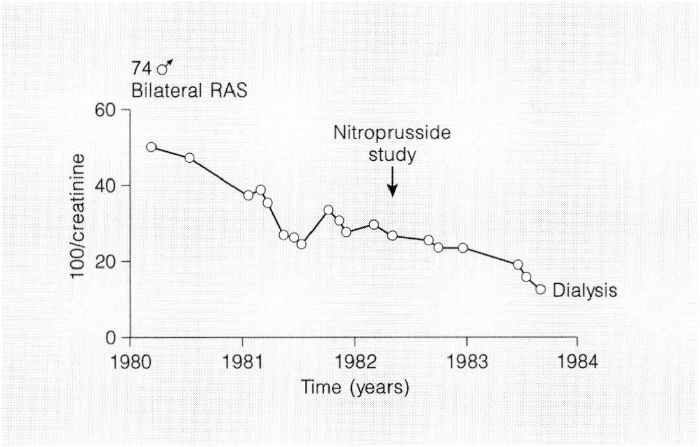

b

Fig. 2. **a** Abrupt fall in renal blood flow (ERPF) and glomerular filtration rates (GFR) during arterial pressure reduction using sodium nitroprusside (NP) in patients with critical bilateral renal artery stenosis. This sensitivity to pressure reduction could be reversed with revascularization of one kidney. [From ref. 7, with permission.] **b** Progressive loss of kidney function (shown as reciprocal creatinine) to ESRD in a patient with critical bilateral renal artery disease (RAS) who was not subjected to revascularization.

Recent studies have focused directly upon detecting high-grade vascular lesions. Studies using duplex ultrasonography applied to patients with advanced renal disease suggest that renovascular lesions may be present in 3 of 21 (14.3%) subjects studied [9]. These estimates are in general agreement with the results of a prospective survey performed in Great Britain [10] in new patients reaching ESRD, of whom 10 of 64 (14%) over age 50 had stenotic renal artery lesions.

These results imply that a substantial fraction of patients reaching ESRD without a specific renal diagnosis may have vascular lesions affecting the kidneys. Such observations raise the possibility that 'ischemic nephropathy' may be a commonly overlooked, reversible cause of ESRD.

Pathophysiology of Progressive Renal Failure

It should be emphasized, however, that identification of vascular disease of the renal arteries does not establish its role in progressive renal failure. Major gaps remain in our understanding of the pathogenesis of renal injury beyond an occlusive vascular lesion, as previously reviewed [11]. Unlike most other organs, the blood supply to the kidney delivers a surplus of oxygen, of which less than 10–15% is required for the metabolic needs of the tissue and for support of tubular reabsorption. Renal venous sampling from underperfused kidneys in humans fails to demonstrate an excess of erythropoietin, leading the authors of another study [12] to question whether tissue ischemia is present. Remarkably, the venous oxygen tension from underperfused kidneys is elevated as compared with the contralateral side [13]. Hence, the assumption that loss of renal viability beyond a vascular stenotic lesion represents an 'ischemic' pathologic lesion based upon deprivation of oxygen may not be precisely correct.

Then by what mechanisms does renal injury develop beyond a chronic vascular lesion? Studies of acute renal failure induced by interruption of the blood supply may not apply directly, but provide a paradigm within which to consider this problem. A full discussion of this issue is beyond the scope of the present paper, but is considered more fully elsewhere [11]. A proposed pathogenic pathway is shown in figure 3.

It is likely that a critical stenotic lesion induces repetitive episodes of reduced renal perfusion. Such episodes lead to localized deficits of adenosine triphosphate derived energy sources within the kidney, allow intracellular calcium entry, and disturb the vascular endothelium sufficiently to release parenchymal mediators of cellular proliferation and fibrosis. These insults foster gradual degradation of the cytoskeleton of renal cells. Transient rises in arterial pressure during daily fluctuations may allow partial recovery, only to be overridden by a repeat episode of hypoperfusion. It should be emphasized that such changes in poststenotic pressure may be magnified by systemic antihypertensive therapy [14].

Unfortunately, little is known that specifically identifies patients with deteriorating renal function who will benefit from renal revascularization. Although the glomerular filtration occasionally improves dramatically, the average glomerular filtration rate after repair of the renal arteries generally changes little [10, 15, 16]. Until specific indicators of renal salvageability are known, some patients will be subjected to renal revascularization with little clinical benefit.

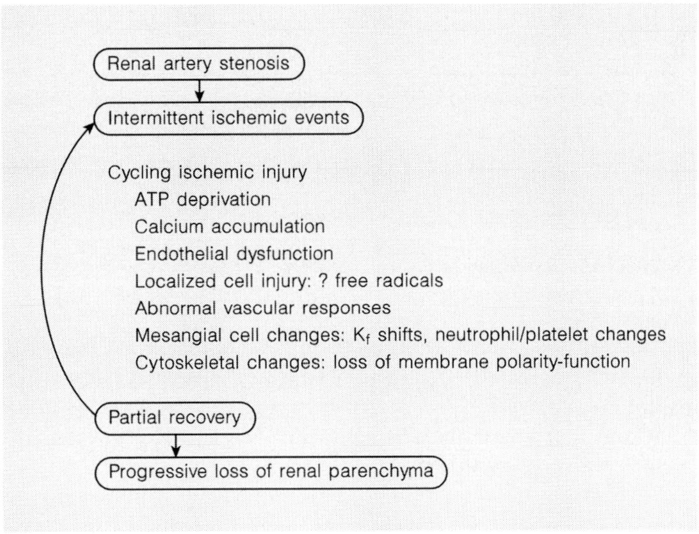

Fig. 3. Schematic paradigm illustrating some of the putative mechanisms by which repetitive hypoperfusion to the kidney beyond a vascular lesion may lead to progressive renal injury. [From ref. 11, with permission.]

Prevalence of Atherosclerotic Disease in ESRD Patients in the US

In 1991, more than 135,000 patients received chronic dialytic support under the ESRD program. The Case = Mix Adequacy of Dialysis Study [1] was undertaken in 1992 to examine a sample of this population in detail. By 1994, this sample reached 7,200 patients for whom details of clinical comorbid data regarding associated medical conditions were known. To estimate the pool of candidates likely to harbor atherosclerotic renovascular disease, we chose to examine data from Caucasian patients above the age of 60 years whose primary renal diagnosis was hypertensive nephrosclerosis. Table 1 shows summary statistics for both Caucasian and African American patients over the age of 60 years. Diabetes was excluded in this category. Coronary artery disease was identified by the presence of angina, prior percutaneous transluminal coronary angioplasty, coronary artery graft, or congestive heart failure. Atherosclerotic peripheral vascular disease (ASPVD) was identified by the presence of extremity amputation, claudication, or loss of distal pulses. Both coronary artery disease and ASPVD were common in all ESRD patients over age 60, but most prevalent in Caucasians with the diagnosis of hypertensive nephrosclerosis. African American patients with ESRD were considered separately, based upon preliminary renal biopsy data during the feasibility phase of the AASK trial, indicating that the vast majority of such individuals indeed had features of nephrosclerosis as the primary renal lesion without other diagnoses [17].

For comparison of comorbid atherosclerotic risk factors in nondialyzed subjects, similar information was obtained during review of 304 azotemic patients (defined as a creatinine concentration ≥2.0 mg/dl undergoing surgical renal revascularization at Mayo Clinic for atherosclerotic renal artery disease. The mean preoperative creatinine value was 3.3 ± 0.4 (range 2.0–10.1) mg/dl. The features of these patients and their comorbid conditions have been described previously [18]. These data are summarized in table 1.

Table 1. Atherosclerotic diseases in the US ESRD population Case-Mix Adequacy of Dialysis Study [1] (%; total n = 7,200)

	Caucasians (≥60 years)		African Americans (≥60 years)		Surgery (hypertension and atherosclerotic renal artery disease)
	hypertension (n = 692)	all other diagnoses (n = 1,552)	hypertension (n = 448)	all other diagnoses (n = 613)	(n = 304)
Coronary artery disease[1]	66.3[a]	58.2	52.7	56	52[c]
Peripheral vascular disease[2]	28.3[b]	25.8	21	29.7	56[c]
Active smoker	12.9	9.4	15.2	10	not available

[a] $p < 0.01$ vs. all other diagnoses; [b] $p < 0.5$ vs. all other diagnoses; [c] $p < 0.01$ vs. ESRD-hypertension (Caucasians).

1 History of coronary artery disease, angina, coronary artery bypass graft, abnormal angiography, percutaneous transluminal coronary angioplasty.

2 Claudication, history of peripheral vascular disease, amputation, absent foot pulses.

The prevalence of clinically evident coronary artery disease ranged from 52 to 67% in all subjects. The highest rates were in ESRD patients with hypertensive nephrosclerosis (67%; $p < 0.01$ vs. all other groups). Clinically manifest ASPVD was present in 21–30% of the subjects reaching ESRD. As might be expected, ASPVD was highly prevalent in the group undergoing revascularization surgery (56%; $p < 0.01$ vs. all ESRD groups). Seventy-five percent underwent aortic replacement at the time of renal revascularization.

Estimated Costs of ESRD Related to Atherosclerotic Renal Disease

Little detailed information is available regarding patients reaching ESRD primarily because of atherosclerotic disease. Using estimates based upon the angiographic literature noted above, we assumed for this analysis that 50% of the Caucasian patients in 1991 with clinical ASPVD above age 60 years with no other specific renal diagnosis may have vascular lesions contributing to the progression to ESRD [5, 19, 20]. Table 2 identifies the potential costs for dialysis services of such individuals at the 1993 level. The costs of dialysis now exceed USD 47,000/year [1]. These estimates suggest that 1.34% of all ESRD patients or 14% of patients over 60 years of age with hypertensive nephrosclerosis have occlusive renal vascular disease. This represents more than 1,800 patients at annual costs of nearly USD 87 million for dialysis services.

How do costs of dialysis care for such patients compare with costs of surgical renal revascularization? Remarkably little information is available either for charges or medical resource costs of such procedures. Summarized in table 2 are figures from 154 azotemic patients whose charges and hospital resource use were reviewed in detail at Mayo Clinic between 1980 and 1993 [Schneider, personal commun.] Charges were adjusted for inflation to the 1993 level, including adjustment for Medicare charge limitations. Diagnostic evaluation including preoperative angiography was not included. As noted, the median inten-

Table 2. Cost estimates for atherosclerotic renal artery disease

Dialysis costs	Patients at risk
Number with ESRD on dialysis (1991 cohort)	135,328
Caucasians ≥60 years (31.1%)	42,987
+ renal diagnosis + hypertension (30.8%)	12,963
+ peripheral vascular disease (28.3%)	3,668
assume 50% with critical renal artery disease	*1,834* dialysis patients
1991 annual dialysis costs, USD	
Medicare payment	38,400
Patient and other sources	8,600
Dialysis costs/patient	*46,900*
Total annual dialysis costs: 1,834 × 46,900	86,014,600

Surgical costs for renal revascularization in azotemic atherosclerotic patients (n = 154)

	Median	Range
Intensive care unit stay, days	4	0–52
Total hospital days	17	3–132
Surgical costs/patient, USD	*38,097*	18,922–308,738

Inflation adjusted to the 1993 level (Mayo Clinic; courtesy of Chris Schneider).

sive care unit stay was 4 days,while the median hospital stay was 17 days. The median charge for this procedure was in excess of USD 38,000. Hence, the charges for surgical renal revascularization in atherosclerotic patients were similar, but somewhat lower than the costs of 1 year's dialysis charge.

Discussion

These observations underscore the high prevalence and costs of atherosclerotic disease in ESRD patients. Review of the comorbid characteristics of ESRD patients presented here indicates that clinical peripheral vascular disease, suggesting advanced aortic atherosclerosis, exceeds 28% in Caucasian patients with the diagnosis of hypertensive nephrosclerosis. Based upon the available literature, we estimated that half of these may have associated renovascular disease. These estimates are in striking concordance with small, prospective surveys of patients with advanced renal failure from the southeastern US and Great Britain [9, 10] in which 14% of the patients over age 50 years had high-grade atherosclerotic occlusion.

Nonetheless, these estimates must be viewed with skepticism. As noted in table 1, nearly 44% of the patients with azotemic atherosclerotic disease and renal failure do not have associated ASPVD with symptoms. From this perspective, the assumptions used here underestimate the prevalence of renovascular disease. Furthermore, critical renovascular disease may occur in patients of other races, ages, and diagnostic categories which are not represented here. Conversely, it is unlikely that renal artery disease detected in patients with ASPVD represents the dominant factor in the progression of renal failure in all such patients. Hence, the true prevalence of 'critical' renal artery disease may be less than stated here. It is likely that these factors largely offset each other. Our estimates for the US dialysis population are supported by the clinical diagnosis of renal vascular disease as a cause for ESRD made by Mailloux et al. [20] in a long-term study of 683 patients entering dialysis in New York over 20 years. In this group, 16% of older Caucasians were identified as having clinical renal vascular disease. Taken together, these data argue that high-grade renal vascular disease is commonly present in patients with hypertension reaching ESRD.

Is renovascular disease a central element in the progression of renal failure in these patients? Can renal revascularizaton reduce the progression to ESRD? The answers to these questions remain unclear. In many cases moderate vascular occlusion without evident hemodynamic effect appears to be only minimally related to the development of ESRD. While critical stenosis can be demonstrated occasionally, no easily performed functional study allows this diagnosis to be made with certainty. There is a pressing need to define more precisely the processes identified in figure 3 which mediate renal parenchymal injury beyond an occlusive vascular lesion. In the final analysis, improvement in renal function following revascularization with angioplasty or surgery is the most compelling verification of critical hemodynamic effects. In most operative series, however, a meaningful *improvement* in kidney function (defined as reduced serum creatinine concentration) is unusual, ranging between 25 and 35% [10, 15, 16, 21–23]. Most often, no change in creatinine is observed. Based upon the logic that atherosclerotic lesions can progress, it is argued that a stable creatinine value represents a positive effect of 'preservation of the renal function' [24]. However, the actual rate of vascular progression of atherosclerotic disease is uncertain and appears to be no greater than 40–45% over 5 years. It may be substantially less [25].

These considerations make more difficult the decision as to whether patients with progressive 'nephrosclerosis' should be screened for renovascular disease and subjected to renal revascularization if stenotic lesions are detected. The present report confirms the high costs, both in terms of hospital resource utilization and actual charges, associated with surgical revascularization of azotemic patients. It should be emphasized that this group had a high rate (75%) of combined aortic and renal procedures. The complexity of hospitalization, resources used, and patient risks increases with combined procedures. Furthermore, risks are closely related to the degree of preoperative renal failure. Unfortunately, patients who stand to gain the most from renal revascularization, specifically those with progressing azotemia, face the highest risks of intervention. Remarkably, the overall costs of surgical intervention may be less than those incurred over the course of 1 year of dialysis therapy (table 2). From that perspective, the societal investment in surgical revascularization may be worthwhile if other considerations were clinically persuasive. As closer examination of the outcomes of medical care increases, considerations of costs will become ever more pressing. These concerns highlight the need for better methods of predicting patient-specific risks and benefits of revascularization, ideally by means of prospective clinical trials.

What are the consequences of *not* pursuing renal revascularization in patients suspected of reaching ESRD on the basis of atherosclerotic renal artery disease? Mailloux et al. [20] have followed patients in this category for nearly 20 years. Such patients have a higher prevalence of widespread atherosclerotic disease than the general dialysis population. As shown in table 1, this figure may be considerable. The overall prognosis of such patients is poor, with survival after 5 years of dialytic therapy <20%. Cardiac events and sudden death accounted for the largest share of deaths, some of which have been attributed to the hemodynamic stresses of hemodialysis. Avoiding such hemodynamic challenge may improve survival, but this has not been proven. Although not directly comparable, azotemic patients undergoing renal revascularization have an improved median survival of more than 4 years [18].

Taken together, the problem of widespread atherosclerotic disease affects an increasing number of patients with ESRD. Prevalence estimates from the USRDS Case-Mix Adequacy of Dialysis Study [1] indicate that approximately 14% of the ESRD patients may have significant renovascular disease as a component of their progressive renal failure. The costs of dialytic care in this group may exceed USD 87 million annually. Improved recognition of the features of renal failure produced by vascular occlusive disease and early intervention merit further research and close attention to improve both survival and quality of life in such patients. Prospective studies to address role and optimal timing of revascularization to preserve renal function in such individuals are urgently needed.

Acknowledgments

Portions of this paper were prepared with data obtained from the US Renal Data System, USRDS 1995 Annual Data Report, The National Institutes of Health, National Institute of Diabetes and Digestive and Kidney Diseases, Bethesda, Md., USA, April 1995.

References

1 National Institutes of Health USRDS 1994 Annual Data Report. Am J Kidney Dis 1994;24(suppl 2): 1–181.

2 Kaylor WM, Novick AC, Ziegelbaum M, Vidt DG: Reversal of end-stage renal failure with surgical revascularization in patients with atherosclerotic renal artery occlusion. J Urol 1989;141:486–488.

3 Scoble JE, Hamilton G: Atherosclerotic renovascular disease: Remediable cause of renal failure in the elderly. Br Med J 1990;300:1670–1671.

4 Hansen KJ: Prevalence of ischemic nephropathy in the atherosclerotic population. Am J Kidney Dis 1994; 24:615–621.

5 Swartbol P, Thorvinger BOT, Parsson H, Norgren L: Renal artery stenosis in patients with peripheral vascular disease and its correlation to hypertension: A retrospective study. Int Angiol 1992;11:195–199.

6 May AG, De Weese JA, Rob CG: Hemodynamic effects of arterial stenosis. Surgery 1963;53:513–524.

7 Textor SC, Novick A, Tarazi RC, Klimas V, Vidt DG, Pohl M: Critical perfusion pressure for renal function in patients with bilateral atherosclerotic renal vascular disease. Ann Intern Med 1985;102:309–314.

8 Textor SC, Smith-Powell L: Poststenotic arterial pressure, renal haemodynamics and sodium excretion during graded pressure reduction in conscious rats with one- and two-kidney coarctation hypertension. J Hypertens 1988;6:311–319.

9 O'Neil EA, Hansen KJ, Canzanello VJ, Pennell TC, Dean RH: Prevalence of ischemic nephropathy in patients with renal insufficiency. Am Surg 1992;58:485–490.

10 Scoble JE, Maher ER, Hamilton G, Dick R, Sweny P, Moorhead JF: Atherosclerotic renovascular disease causing renal impairment: A case for treatment. Clin Nephrol 1989;31: 119–122.

11 Textor SC: Pathophysiology of renal failure in ischemic nephropathy. Am J Kidney Dis 1994;24:642–651.

12 Wiecek A, Kokot F, Kuczera M, Grzesszczak W, Kierstztejn M: Plasma erythropoietin concentration in renal venous blood of patients with unilateral renovascular hypertension. Nephrol Dial Transplant 1992; 7:221–224.

13 Nielsen K, Rehling M, Henriksen JH: Renal vein oxygen saturation in renal artery stenosis. Clin Physiol 1992;12:179–184.
14 Textor SC, Novick AC, Steinmuller DR, Streem SB: Renal failure limiting antihypertensive therapy as an indication for renal revascularization. Arch Intern Med 1983;143: 2208–2211.
15 Englund R, Brown MA: Renal angioplasty for renovascular disease: A reappraisal. J Cardiovasc Surg 1991; 32:76–80.
16 Mercier C, Piquet P, Alimi Y, Tournigand P, Albrand J: Occlusive disease of the renal arteries and chronic renal failure: The limits of reconstructive surgery. Ann Vasc Surg 1990;4:166–170.
17 Fogo A, Smith MC, Cleaveland W, Debruge J, Agodoa L, AASK Pilot Investigators: Renal biopsy findings in the African-American Study of Kidney Disease (AASK). J Am Soc Nephrol 1994;5:560.
18 Hallett JW, Textor SC, Kos PB, Nicpon G, Bower TC, Cherry KJ, Glovicski P, Pairolero PC: Advanced renovascular hypertension and renal insufficiency: Trends in medical comorbidity and surgical approach from 1970 to 1993. J Vasc Surg 1995;21:750–759.
19 Valentine RJ, Clagett GP, Miller GL, Myers SI, Martin JD, Chervu A: The coronary risk of unsuspected renal artery stenosis. J Vasc Surg 1993;18:433–439.
20 Mailloux LU, Napolitano B, Bellucci AG, Vernace M, Wilkes BM, Mossey RT: Renal vascular disease causing end-stage renal disease: Incidence, clinical correlates, and outcomes. A 20-year clinical experience. Am J Kidney Dis 1994;24: 622–629.
21 Hallett JW, Fowl R, O'Brien PC, Bernatz PE, Pairolero PC, Cherry KJ, Hollier LH: Renovascular operations in patients with chronic renal insufficiency: Do the benefits justify the risks? J Vasc Surg 1987;5:622–627.
22 Tarazi RY, Hertzer NR, Beven EG, O'Hara PJ, Anton GE, Krajewski LP: Simultaneous aortic reconstruction and renal revascularization: Risk factors and late results in eighty-nine patients. J Vasc Surg 1987;5:707–714.
23 Hansen KJ, Starr SM, Sands RE, Burkart JM, Plonk GW, Dean RH: Contemporary surgical management of renovascular disease. J Vasc Surg 1992;16:319–330.
24 Novick AC: Management of renovascular disease: A surgical perspective. Circulation 1991;83(suppl 1): 167–171.
25 Pohl MA, Horner C, Goormastic M, Novick A: Does renal revascularization preserve renal function in patients with atherosclerotic renal artery stenosis? An ongoing prospective study. J Am Soc Nephrol 1991; 2:242.

Blood Purification

Blood Purif 1996;14:315–320

Steven J. Rosansky

Medical Service, Dorn Veterans Hospital, and Department of Internal Medicine, University of South Carolina School of Medicine, Columbia, S.C., USA

Treatment of Hypertension in Renal Failure Patients: When Do We Overtreat? When Do We Undertreat?

Key Words

Dialysis, survival
Hypertension
Renal failure

Abstract

Despite the commonplace nature of hypertension in chronic dialysis patients, many issues remain unresolved. According to current JNC/V (see text) recommendations, a systolic blood pressure of < 120 mm Hg is optimal, 120–129 mm Hg is normal, and one of 130–139 mm Hg is high-normal. The majority of dialysis patients receiving treatment in the United States is probably not maintained in the optimal blood pressure range. However, if the J curve hypothesis has credence, many of our dialysis patients may be susceptible to overtreatment, especially of their diastolic blood pressure. In patients with ischemic cardiovascular disease, several studies show a decrease in survival with diastolic blood pressures < 85 mm Hg. This J curve phenomenon is seen predominantly in patients with ischemic heart disease. Since many, and possibly most, of the currently treated end-stage renal disease patients in the United States have existing atherosclerotic cardiovascular disease when they start chronic dialysis therapy, lowering of the diastolic blood pressure below a J threshold may be dangerous. This problem may be especially prevalent in diabetics with diabetic cardiomyopathy. Diabetics and other end-stage renal disease patients may be started on hemodialysis with glomerular filtration rates in the 10- to 15-cm^3/min range. Patients with high residual renal function may have small intradialytic weight gains and frequent intradialytic hypotension. This 'overtreatment' may lead to postdialysis arrhythmias and sudden death in chronic dialysis patients. As in the nonrenal failure population, end-stage renal disease patients with left ventricular hypertrophy have a 2- to 3-fold increased risk of death from cardiovascular diseases, and all cause mortality. In contrast to nonrenal failure patients, normotensive ESRD patients may show an increase of left ventricular mass over time. Although left ventricular hypertrophy can be reversed with good blood pressure control, patients are often undertreated based on analysis of dialysis clinic blood pressures. Even if clinic systolic blood pressure levels are optimal, chronic dialysis patients may still have unacceptably high ambulatory blood pressure levels due to a rise in nocturnal blood pressure with sleep.

KARGER

E-Mail karger@karger.ch
Fax + 41 61 306 12 34
http://www.karger.ch

0253–5068/96/0144–0315$10.00/0

Steven J. Rosansky, MD
Department of Veterans Affairs
Willliam Jennings Bryan Dorn Veterans Hospital
6439 Garners Ferry Road
Columbia, SC 29209–1639 (USA)

The importance of hypertension as a national public health issue is well accepted. Most renal physicians are well versed in hypertension diagnosis and treatment. Many, if not most, of the chronic dialysis patients are currently receiving antihypertensive therapy. Despite the commonplace nature of hypertension, in chronic dialysis patients, many issues remain unresolved.

According to current JNC/V recommendations [1] a systolic blood pressure of <120 mm Hg is optimal, one of 120–129 mm Hg is normal, and a systolic blood pressure of 130–139 mm Hg is high-normal [1]. My guess is that the vast majority of dialysis patients receiving treatment in the United States are maintained beyond the optimal or normal blood pressure level, and probably most are beyond the high-normal level as defined by JNC/V. On the other hand, if the J curve hypothesis has credence, many of our dialysis patients may be susceptible to overtreatment, especially of their diastolic blood pressure [2].

Systolic Blood Pressure versus Adjusted Coronary Heart Disease Death Rate

The MRFIT study [3] is the largest available prospective data on the relationship between blood pressure levels and ischemic heart disease risk in middle-aged American men. This study screened almost 350,000 men 35–37 years of age and followed this cohort for approximately 12 years. These men were not previously hospitalized for a myocardial infarction and were much healthier than the prototype patient of the US end-stage renal disease (ESRD) population. The MRFIT study showed a clear, strong, continuous relationship between systolic blood pressure levels and coronary heart disease events even after controlling for other risk factors related to coronary heart disease. Even at a systolic blood pressure of 120–129 mm Hg, the relative risk for coronary heart disease events, as compared with those subjects with a systolic blood pressure <110 mm Hg, was 1.32:1.

Left Ventricular Hypertrophy (LVH) versus Survival

Several studies have established a relationship between echorcardiographically determined LVH and risk of death from cardiovascular disease [4]. This risk is approximately 2–3 times the risk in patients without LVH. Although LVH can be reversed with hypertension treatment, this reversal has not been shown to improve survival beyond that due to blood pressure control. In addition, hypertension control may explain only 25% of the regression of LVH with blood pressure treatment [5].

LVH in the ESRD Dialysis Population

As in the nonrenal failure population, ESRD patients with LVH have a 2- to 3-fold increased risk of death from cardiovascular diseases, and all cause mortality [6]. In contrast to nonrenal failure patients, normotensive ESRD patients may show an increase of left ventricular mass over time [7]. This increase may result from uncontrolled anemia, but may also be due to increased collagen fiber deposition between myocardial cells (intramyocardiocytic fibrosis) [8]. This nonmyocyte increase in left ventricular mass may be very prevalent in the chronic dialysis patient. Despite the possible occurrence of irreversible left ventricular collagen deposition as a cause of LVH in dialysis patients, Cannella et al. [9]

demonstrated that LVH can be reversed with good blood pressure control in this population.

What Is the Published Evidence of Hypertension Undertreatment in the Current Dialysis Population?

Cheigh et al. [10, 11] published two studies depicting 24-hour monitored blood pressure results in hemodialysis and chronic peritoneal dialysis patients, respectively. Blood pressure control in these patients was poor, with 58% of the patients having an uncontrolled systolic blood pressure (mean >150 mm Hg) and 39% an uncontrolled diastolic blood pressure (>90 mm Hg). Data on mean pre- and post-dialysis blood pressure levels in large cohorts of chronic dialysis patients have not yet been published; nevertheless, even if dialysis blood pressure levels are <140 mm Hg before and after dialysis, chronic dialysis patients may still have unacceptably high blood pressure levels due to their abnormal circadian blood pressure profile. We have reported absence of a decline or a rise in nocturnal blood pressure with sleep in chronic dialysis patients [12]. Thus, analysis of clinic blood pressures in dialysis patients without 24-hour blood pressure monitoring may provide a falsely favorable picture. Also, if one looks at mean blood pressure in a chronic dialysis population, one may get a falsely low level due to low blood pressures in many patients who were hypertensive and became normotensive or hypotensive towards the end of their lives on chronic dialysis.

Does Blood Pressure Control Affect Mortality in Chronic Dialysis Patients?

Rostand et al. [13] were able to demonstrate a relationship, although a weak one, between diastolic blood pressure prior to the onset of hemodialysis treatment and ischemic heart disease events. More recently, Tomita et al. [14] showed that the mean systolic blood pressure prior to dialysis sessions was significantly higher in 9 patients who died within 3 years of introduction to dialysis versus survivors at the 3-year interval. Zager et al. [unpubl. data] looked at mean pre- and postdialysis blood pressures and their relationship to the next year's chronic dialysis patient survival. These authors found that each 1-mm Hg increase in systolic blood pressure was associated with a 3% increase in the risk of death the following year. Charra et al. [15] demonstrated excellent survival of young chronic renal failure patients whose blood pressures were controlled without antihypertensive medications. These patients were dialyzed 8 h per treatment three times per week utilizing a 1-m^2/Kiil parallel-plate dialyzer. Charra et al. [15] attributed the excellent survival in this patient population to slow dialysis with excellent nonpharmacological blood pressure control.

Can Blood Pressure Be Controlled by Ultrafiltration Alone?

In contrast to the results reported by Charra et al. [15], other nephrologists do not find this close relationship between ultrafiltration and control of blood pressure. For example, Cheigh et al. [10] found that only 50% of their chronically dialyzed patients had a decline of the blood pressure with ultrafiltration during dialysis. Interestingly, approximately 70% of the African American subjects had a decline of the blood pressure with ultrafiltration as compared with only 28% of their Caucasian patients. In addition, several studies support the view that blood pressure does not relate to intradialytic weight gain. Kooman et al. [16] found that the 24-hour blood pressure was not different when measured 1 or 2 days after dialysis treatment.

Overtreatment of Hypertension

Although most studies to date show an improvement in survival with a lower systolic blood pressure, the same cannot be said for the diastolic blood pressure. Although the JNC/V [1] recommends a diastolic blood pressure of <80 mm Hg as optimal, this may not be an appropriate level for some patients.

In patients with ischemic cardiovascular disease, several studies show a decrease in survival with diastolic blood pressures <85 mm Hg. This J curve phenomenon is predominantly seen in patients with ischemic heart disease. Farnett et al. [17] reviewed 13 major hypertension treatment trials. These authors found a J curve in 10 of the 13 published studies with a nadir at 84 mm Hg. Alderman et al. [18] showed that too small (<6 mm Hg) or too large (>18 mm Hg) a change in diastolic blood pressure was associated with an increased risk of a myocardial infarction. Many studies that show this J curve relationship demonstrate a continuous improved survival with lower diastolic blood pressures if patients with coronary artery disease are excluded from the analysis.

Since many, and possibly most, of the currently treated ESRD patients in the United States have existing atherosclerotic cardiovascular disease when they start chronic dialysis therapy, lowering of diastolic blood pressure below a J threshold may be dangerous. This may be especially hazardous for those ESRD patients with increased left ventricular mass and decreased left ventricular compliance. As a result of the decreased compliance associated with increased left ventricular mass, ultrafiltration during dialysis may decrease the left ventricular preload and may result in intradialytic hypotension. This hypotension may stimulate coronary ischemia and possibly postdialysis arrhythmias. According to Ritz et al. [19], this problem may be especially prevalent in diabetics with diabetic cardiomyopathy. This cardiomyopathy may be due to a combination of uremia and diabetes-related myocardial interstitial fibrosis. This extensive fibrosis may predispose to electrical instability with increased reentrant arrhythmias and sudden death. This pathophysiologic process may be exacerbated by intradialytic hypotension.

Overtreatment Hypothesis for Hemodialysis Patients

Currently, diabetics compose approximately 30% of the US ESRD population. According to a recent US Renal Data System survey, diabetics in the US are often started on hemodialysis with glomerular filtration rates in the 10- to 15-ml/min range. If patients with a high residual renal function have greater urine outputs than those with minimal residual renal function, this may lead to smaller intradialytic weight gains in those patients with greater urine outputs. These smaller weight gains may result in greater obligatory removal of fluid (below dry body weight) with more frequent intradialytic hypotension as compared with patients with minimal residual renal function.

This 'overtreatment' may lead to postdialysis arrhythmias and sudden death in chronic dialysis patients by the following mechanisms (fig. 1): Hypertension may result in an in-

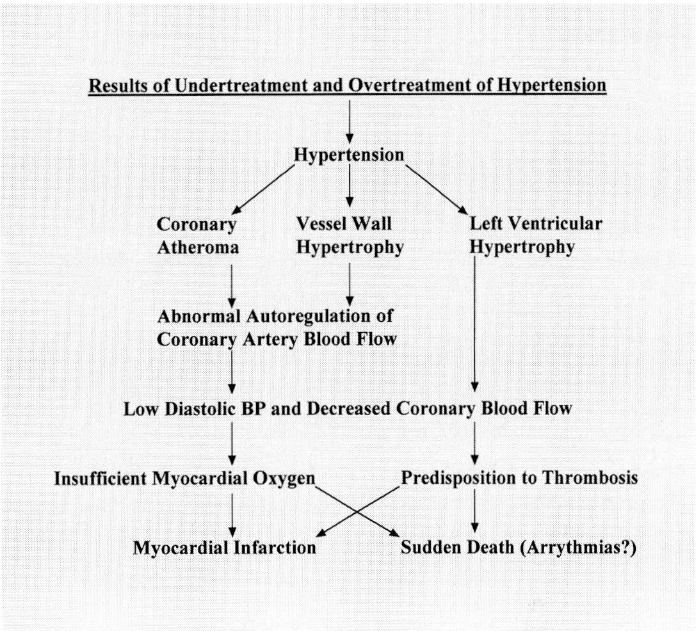

Fig. 1. How hypertension undertreatment may lead to coronary atheroma, vessel wall hypertrophy, and abnormal autoregulation of coronary blood flow is shown. Under these conditions, overaggressive lowering of the diastolic blood pressure may lead to sudden death caused by myocardial ischemia and infarction and ventricular arrhythmias.

creased tendency to atherosclerosis. Hypertension may also cause coronary artery vessel wall hypertrophy. Both of these processes may lead to abnormal autoregulation of coronary artery blood flow. In addition, hypertension may promote further hypertrophy of the myocardial ventricular wall. These factors taken together may result (especially during intradialytic hypotension) in coronary ischemia with resultant arrhythmias and sudden death. In addition, chronic hypotension during and after dialysis sessions may lead to asymptomatic cerebral ischemia and renal ischemia with loss of residual renal function.

Conclusion

Although nephrologists are well aware of the need for hypertension treatment and control in chronic dialysis patients, the goal blood pressure of this population needs to be arrived at through prospective studies which evaluate the effects of high or low blood pressure levels on the chronic dialysis population.

Acknowledgments

I gratefully acknowledge the assistance with medical references by Charletta Felder and the assistance with manuscript preparation by Ann Martin, Michael R. Littlejohn, and Khoa N. Vo.

References

1 Joint National Committee on Detection, Evaluation, and Treatment of High Blood Pressure: 5th Report of the Joint National Committee on Detection, Evaluation, and Treatment of High Blood Pressure. Bethesda, National Institutes of Health, 1993.

2 Fletcher AE, Bulpitt CJ: How far should blood pressure be lowered? N Engl J Med 1992;326:251–254.

3 Stamler J, Stamler R, Neaton JD: Blood pressure, systolic and diastolic, and cardiovascular risks. US population data. Arch Intern Med 1993; 153:598–615.

4 Levy D, Garrison RJ, Savage DD, Kannel WB, Castelli WP: Prognostic implications of echocardiographically determined left ventricular mass in the Framingham Heart Study. N Engl J Med 1990;322: 1561–1566.

5 Dahlof B, Pennert K, Hansson L: Reversal of left ventricular hypertrophy in hypertensive patients: A meta-analysis of 109 treatment studies. Am J Hypertens 1992;5:95–110.

6 Silberberg JS, Barre PE, Prichard SS, Sniderman AD: Impact of left ventricular hypertrophy on survival in end-stage renal disease. Kidney Int 1989;36:286–290.

7 Huting J, Kramer W, Schutterle G, Wizemann V: Analysis of left-ventricular changes associated with chronic hemodialysis: A noninvasive follow-up study. Nephron 1988; 49:284–290.

8 Mall G, Huther W, Schneider J, Lundin P, Ritz E: Diffuse intermyocardiocytic fibrosis in uremic patients. Nephrol Dial Transplant 1990;5:39–44.

9 Cannella G, Paoletti E, Delfino R, Peloso G, Molinari S, Traverso GB: Regression of left ventricular hypertrophy in hypertensive dialyzed uremic patients on long-term antihypertensive therapy. Kidney Int 1993;44:881–886.

10 Cheigh JS, Milite C, Sullivan JF, Rubin AL, Stenzel KH: Hypertension is not adequately controlled in hemodialysis patients. Am J Kidney Dis 1992;19:453–459.

11 Cheigh JS, Serur D, Paguirigan M, Stenzel KH, Rubin A: How well is hypertension controlled in CAPD patients? Adv Perit Dial 1994;10: 55–58.

12 Rosansky SJ, Johnson KL, Hutchinson C, Erdel S: Blood pressure changes during daytime sleep and comparison of daytime and nighttime sleep-related blood pressure changes in patients with chronic renal failure. J Am Soc Nephrol 1993; 4:1172–1177.

13 Rostand SG, Kirk KA, Rutsky EA: Relationship of coronary risk factors to hemodialysis-associated ischemic heart disease. Kidney Int 1982;22: 304–308.

14 Tomita J, Kimura G, Inoue T, Inenaga T, Sanai T, Kawano Y, Nakamura S, Baba S, Matsuoka H, Omae T: Role of systolic blood pressure in determining prognosis of hemodialyzed patients. Am J Kidney Dis 1995;25:205–212.

15 Charra B, Calemard E, Ruffet M, Chazot C, Terrat JC, Vanel T, Laurent G: Survival as an index of adequacy of dialysis. Kidney Int 1992; 41:1286–1291.

16 Kooman JP, Gladziwa U, Bocker G, Wijnen JA, Bortel L, Luik AJ, de Leeuw PW, van Hoff JP, Leunissen KM: Blood pressure during the interdialytic period in hemodialysis patients: Estimation of representative blood pressure values. Nephrol Dial Transplant 1992;7:917–923.

17 Farnett L, Mulrow CD, Linn WD, Lucey CR, Tuley MR: The J-curve phenomenon and the treatment of hypertension: Is there a point beyond which pressure reduction is dangerous? JAMA 1991;265:498–495.

18 Alderman MH, Ooi WL, Madhavan S, Cohen H: Treatment-induced blood pressure reduction and the risk of myocardial infarction. JAMA 1989;262:920–924.

19 Ritz E, Strumpf C, Katz F, Wing AJ, Quellhorst E: Hypertension and cardiovascular risk factors in hemodialyzed diabetic patients. Hypertension 1985;7:118–124.

Blood Purification

Blood Purif 1996;14:321–326

Patrick S. Parfrey
Robert N. Foley

Division of Nephrology,
Health Sciences Centre,
St. John's, Nfld., Canada

Ischemic Heart Disease in Chronic Uremia

Abstract

The burden of ischemic heart disease is high in dialysis patients. Ischemia may result from atherosclerotic and nonatherosclerotic disease and may cause myocardial infarction and angina. The impact of diminished perfusion is intricately associated with the underlying cardiomyopathy, both of which predispose to heart failure. The etiology of ischemia is complex and associated with the underlying cardiomyopathy, whether it be concentric left ventricular hypertrophy, left ventricular dilatation, or systolic dysfunction. Hypertension, diabetes, dyslipidemia, abnormalities of divalent ion metabolism, hypoalbuminemia, and left ventricular hypertrophy are probably adverse risk factors for ischemia, but the relative importance of each is unknown.

Key Words

Cardiomyopathy
Coronary artery disease
End-stage renal disease
Ischemic heart disease

Ischemic heart disease occurs frequently in dialysis patients. A history of myocardial infarction or angina was obtained in 34% of the patients on starting end-stage renal dialysis therapy [1]. The probability of developing myocardial infarction or angina requiring hospitalization following the initiation of dialysis was 10% per year [2]. Although most patients who develop symptoms of ischemic heart disease while on dialysis have had manifestations of disease prior to starting dialysis, 9% develop de novo symptoms of ischemia following initiation of dialysis [3].

Ischemic heart disease results from atherosclerotic disease in the majority of dialysis patients, but in 27% ischemic symptoms were caused by nonatherosclerotic disease [4].

Pathophysiology

In atherosclerotic coronary artery disease, critical stenoses of the coronary arteries result in symptoms of ischemia. In nonatherosclerotic disease symptoms occur in the absence of critical coronary artery disease and result from a reduction in coronary vasodilator reserve, altered myocardial oxygen delivery and use, and small coronary artery disease [5].

In chronic uremia cardiomyopathy may be manifest as concentric left ventricular (LV) hypertrophy, LV dilatation, or systolic dysfunction [6, 7]. LV pressure overload from systemic hypertension or, occasionally, aortic stenosis causes concentric LV hypertrophy. LV volume overload results from anemia, arteriovenous fistula, or blood volume expansion. When LV dilatation occurs [8], compensatory LV hypertrophy develops to maintain the LV wall tension. This type of LV hypertro-

KARGER

E-Mail karger@karger.ch
Fax + 41 61 306 12 34
http://www.karger.ch

0253–5068/96/0144–0321$10.00/0

Dr. Patrick S. Parfrey
Division of Nephrology
Health Sciences Centre
St. John's, Nfld. A1B 3V6 (Canada)

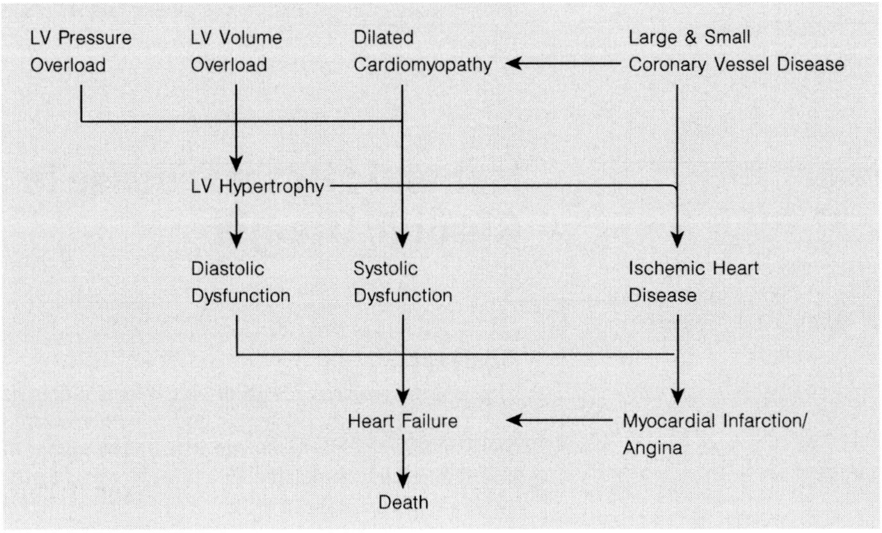

Fig. 1. Relationships between coronary disease, LV hypertrophy, and clinical manifestations of cardiac disease.

phy is termed eccentric hypertrophy. In systolic dysfunction, perhaps resulting from myocyte death, LV dilatation and concomitant LV hypertrophy are often observed. In addition to myocyte hypertrophy, fibroblastic proliferation occurs, leading to intermyocardiocytic fibrosis [9]. Thus, whether cardiomyopathy is manifest as concentric LV hypertrophy, LV dilatation, or systolic dysfunction, LV hypertrophy is characteristic of dialysis patients and is associated with an increased demand for oxygen. LV hypertrophy predisposes to ischemic symptoms, whether such ischemia results from large or small coronary vessel disease. As the demand for oxygen increases, the coronary vasculature dilates above basal, and a further increase in myocardial oxygen requirement may not be met with an adequate increase in coronary flow, especially if there are pathologic changes in the large or small coronary vessels. In coronary artery stenosis, during hyperemia, flow progressively decreases when the degree of stenosis is above 40% and does not differ significantly from basal flow when the stenosis is 80% or greater [10].

Ischemia, whether from large or small vessel coronary disease, predisposes to myocardial dysfunction. In the presence of LV hypertrophy, myocyte death induced by ischemia may be catastrophic, predisposing to LV dilatation and eventually to systolic dysfunction. Both systolic and diastolic dysfunctions predispose to heart failure, with symptoms of pulmonary edema. Thus, diminished perfusion and LV hypertrophy are associated not only with symptoms of ischemia, but also with those of LV muscle dysfunction (fig. 1).

Prognosis

Patients with ischemic heart disease on starting dialysis have a higher mortality rate than those without, the median survival in the former being 44 months and in the latter 56 months [3]. However, this effect is not independent of that due to heart failure. Patients with ischemic heart disease have a similar survival to those without, when survival is corrected for differences in age, diabetes, and heart failure present at baseline [3]. This implies that the adverse impact of ischemic heart disease is mediated via LV muscle dysfunction rather than other effects of decreased perfusion.

Diagnosis

One of the difficulties in studying ischemic heart disease in chronic uremia is determining the role of large versus small vessel coronary disease in causing adverse outcomes. Nonatherosclerotic disease may be the cause of ischemic symptoms in a substantial minority of patients with ischemic heart disease [4]. Furthermore, silent ischemia may be present, particularly in diabetic patients [11]. Many of the noninvasive tests which detect regional hypoperfusion have a low sensitivity and a low specificity for coronary artery disease in dialysis patients [5]. Recently data from the Cleveland Clinic suggest that dobutamine echocardiography may be an adequate diagnostic tool to detect coronary artery disease in dialysis patients [12]. However, this conclusion requires confirmation from larger numbers of patients, tested in different centres. Until this has occurred, the gold standard for the diagnosis of coronary artery disease remains coronary arteriography.

In epidemiological studies, it is clearly impossible to perform coronary arteriography in all subjects. Consequently, ischemic disease can only be defined by the presence of symptoms caused by ischemia: myocardial infarction and angina. This limitation should be borne in mind when assessing risk factors for ischemic heart disease, as it is possible that the risk factors for large vessel coronary disease are different from those causing nonatherosclerotic disease.

Etiology

Atherosclerotic Disease

Multiple factors contribute to the vascular pathology of chronic uremia, including injury to the vessel wall, prothrombotic factors, lipoprotein interactions, and proliferation of smooth muscle [13]. There is evidence of chronic in vivo endothelial activation and injury in uremia [14]. Many hemodialysis patients have normal lipid profiles, but peritoneal dialysis patients may have higher plasma triglyceride and low-density lipoprotein (LDL) levels [13]. Perhaps more important than absolute changes in lipoprotein lipid and apoprotein concentrations is the impact of lipoprotein compositional abnormalities. Dialysis patients have a severe defect in postprandial lipoprotein metabolism which exposes the vascular wall to high chylomicron remnant concentrations [15]. Furthermore, patients on hemodialysis have elevated intermediate-density lipoprotein levels, heterogeneity in the distribution of LDL and apoprotein-specific high-density lipoprotein (HDL) subpopulations, and abnormalities in size and composition of both LDL and HDL [16]. In addition, LDL from uremic patients appears to be more susceptible to in vitro and in vivo oxidation as compared with control subjects [17]. Modification of the recognition of LDL by cells may occur in hemodialysis patients [18]. In hemodialysis patients with or without diabetes mellitus, the serum lipoprotein(a) levels are higher than in normal controls [19, 20].

The adverse impact of hypercholesterolemia in dialysis patients may be confounded by the higher mortality of hypocholesterolemia, associated with malnutrition. The prognostic impact of lipoprotein remnants, oxidized LDL, or altered lipoproteins has not been reported in chronic uremia. In a prospective study of diabetic patients on hemodialysis, those subsequently dying from myocardial in-

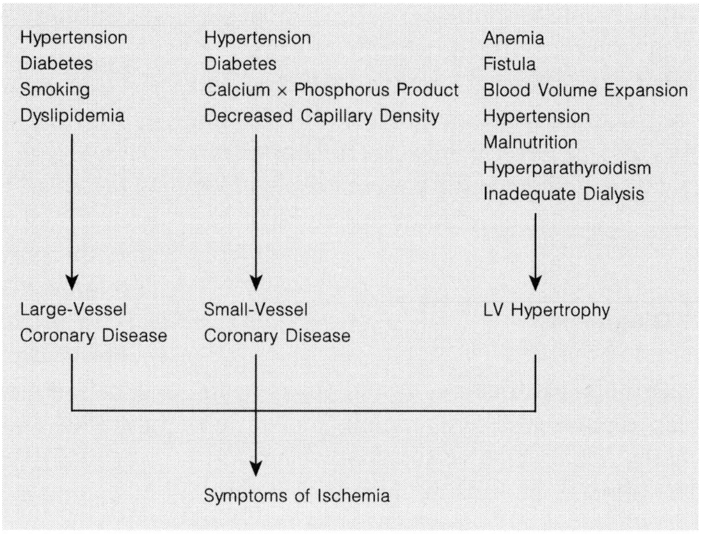

Fig. 2. Etiology of ischemic heart disease.

farction had significantly higher median cholesterol levels than survivors and higher LDL cholesterol levels, LDL:HDL ratios, and apolipoprotein B concentrations [21]. In a second prospective study of 91 chronic dialysis patients [22], high levels of LDL cholesterol were associated with coronary and cerebrovascular events. A third longitudinal study [23] demonstrated that lipoprotein(a) was an independent predictor of fatal events attributable to cardiovascular disease in hemodialysis patients.

Small-Vessel Coronary Disease

In LV hypertrophy small-vessel smooth muscle hypertrophy and endothelial abnormalities occur [24]; these can diminish the coronary reserve. Calcification of small vessels may have a similar effect. The calcium × phosphorus product has been reported to be significantly elevated in symptomatic end-stage renal disease patients without significant coronary artery disease as compared with those with significant lesions [25]. Diabetic patients may have small coronary artery abnormalities with endothelial proliferation, subendothelial fibrosis, exudative deposits of hyaline in the intima, and atheromatous thickening with cholesterol clefts and hyalinized intima [26]. When matched for LV weight and blood pressure level, length and surface density of capillaries in the heart of uremic rats are significantly more reduced than in rats with Goldblatt hypertension [27].

Susceptibility to myocardial ischemia may further increase by dysregulation of high-energy phosphate compounds during ischemia. A reduced phosphocreatine: adenosine 5′-triphosphate ratio under hypoxic stress has been observed in the myocardium of uremic animals [28]. Hyperparathyroidism plays a critical role in the genesis of impaired energy production, transfer, and utilization by the myocardium [29] and thus increases the susceptibility to ischemia.

LV Hypertrophy

The characteristic observation of LV hypertrophy in dialysis patients presumably predisposes to ischemia through the reduction in coronary reserve caused by increased LV muscle mass. In addition to the prevalenc of hypertension, anemia, fistula formation, and blood volume expansion, all of which predispose to LV hypertrophy, malnutrition, hyperparathyroidism, inadequate dialysis, and coronary vessel disease may induce myocyte death [7]. In the presence of LV hypertrophy this cell death may lead to LV dilatation and further adaptive hypertrophy necessary to maintain LV wall tension.

The relative importance of each potential etiological mechanism for ischemic heart disease is unknown (fig. 2). In a prospective study [3] one fifth of the patients had an episode of ischemic heart disease while on dialysis, one half of which were de novo episodes. Older age, diabetes, smoking, hypertension, hypoalbuminemia, and hypocalcemia were all independently associated with the development of de novo ischemic heart disease [3, 30]. Hypocalcemia induces hyperparathyroidism which may produce disturbances in lipid metabolism [31], but probably of more importance is the parathyroid hormone induced intracellular calcium overload that results in derangements of myocardial bioenergetics [29].

In the prospective study described above [3] anemia was not identified as an independent risk factor for the development of de novo ischemic heart disease. This is somewhat surprising as one would expect anemia to decrease the coronary vasodilator reserve. It is likely that the role of anemia will be clarified by trials of erythropoietin therapy in which patients with ischemic heart disease are randomly allocated to either normalization of hemoglobin level or to partial correction of anemia. In fact, partial correction of anemia with erythropoietin reduced exercise-induced myocardial ischemia in dialysis patients with coronary artery disease [32].

Conclusions

The burden of ischemic heart disease is high in dialysis patients. It may result from atherosclerotic and nonatherosclerotic disease. The etiology of ischemia is complex and associated with the underlying cardiomyopathy. Hypertension, diabetes, dyslipidemia, abnormalities of divalent ion metabolism, hypoalbuminemia, and LV hypertrophy are probably adverse risk factors for ischemia, but the relative importance of each is unknown. Frequent adverse clinical outcomes include myocardial infarction, angina, and particularly heart failure.

References

1 Foley RN, Parfrey PS, Hefferton D, Singh I, Simms A, Barret BJ: Advance prediction of early death in patients starting maintenance dialysis. Am J Kidney Dis 1994;23:836–845.

2 Churchill DN, Taylor DW, Cook RJ, la Plante P, Barre P, Cartier P, Fay W, Goldstein M, Jindal K, Mandin H, et al: Canadien Hemodialysis Morbidity Study. Am J Kidney Dis 1992;19:214–234.

3 Parfrey PS, Foley RN, Harnett JD, Kent GM, Murray DC, Barre PE: Ischemic heart disease in chronic uremia. Kidney Int, in press.

4 Rostand SG, Kirk KA, Rutsky EA: Dialysis-associated ischemic heart disease: Insights from coronary angiography. Kidney Int 1984;25:653–659.

5 Rostand SG, Rutsky EA: Ischemic heart disease in chronic renal failure: Demography, epidemiology and pathogenesis; in Parfrey PS, Harnett JD (eds): Cardiac Dysfunction in Chronic Uremia. Boston, Kluwer, 1992, pp 53–66.

6 Parfrey PS, Harnett JD, Foley RN: Heart failure and ischemic heart disease in chronic uremia. Curr Opin Nephrol Hypertens 1995;4:105–110.

7 Parfrey PS, Foley RN, Harnett JD, Kent GM, O'Dea R, Murray DC, Barre PE: Left ventricular disorders in chronic uremia. Nephrol Dial Transplant, in press.

8 London GM, Fabiani F, Marchais SK, de Vernejoul M-C, Guerin AP, Safar ME, Metivier F, Llach F: Uremic cardiomyopathy: An inadequate left ventricular hypertrophy. Kidney Int 1987;31:973–980.

9 Mall G, Huter W, Schneider J, Lundin P, Ritz E: Diffuse intermyocardiocytic fibrosis in uremic patients. Nephrol Dial Transplant 1990;5: 39–44.

10 Uren NG, Melin JA, DeBruyne B, Winjns W, Baudhuin T, Camici PG: Relation between myocardial blood flow and the severity of coronary artery stenosis. N Engl J Med 1993; 330:1782–1788.

11 Jensen T, Borch-Johnsen K, Kofoed-Enerold A, Deckert T: Coronary heart disease in young type 1 (insulin dependent) diabetic patients with and without diabetic nephropathy: Incidence and risk factors. Diabetologia 1987;30:144–148.

12 Albanese J, Nally J, Marwick T, D'Houdt A-M, Wijins W, Vanypersile C: Dobutamine echocardiography is effective in the non-invasive detection of prognostically important coronary artery disease in patients with end-stage renal disease (abstract). J Am Soc Nephrol 1994; 5:322.

13 Shapiro J: Atherogenesis in chronic renal failure; in Parfrey PS, Harnett JD (eds): Cardiac Dysfunction in Chronic Uremia. Boston, Kluwer, 1992, pp 187–204.

14 Gris J-C, Branger B, Vecina F, Al Sabadani B, Fourcadi J, Schred J-F: Increased cardiovascular risk factors and features of endothelial activation and dysfunction in dialyzed uremic patients. Kidney Int 1994; 46:807–813.

15 Weintraub M, Burstein A, Rassin T, Liron M, Ringel Y, Cabili S, Blum M, Peer G, Irina A: Severe defect in clearing postprandial chylomicron remnants in dialysis patients. Kidney Int 1992;42:1247–1252.

16 Joven J, Vilella E, Ahmed S, Cheung MC, Brunzell JD: Lipoprotein heterogeneity in end stage renal disease. Kidney Int 1993;43:410–418.

17 Maggi E, Bellazzi R, Falaschi F, Frattoni A, Perani G, Finardi G, Gazo A, Nai M, Romanini D, Bellomo G: Enhanced LDL oxidation in uremic patients: An additional mechanism for accelerated artherosclerosis? Kidney Int 1994;45:876–883.

18 Reade V, Tailleux A, Reade R, Harduin P, Cachera C, Tacquet A, Fruchart J-C, Fievet C: Expression of apolipoprotein B epitopes in low density lipoproteins of hemodialyzed patients. Kidney Int 1993;44: 1360–1365.

19 Hirata K, Kikuchi S, Saku K, Jimi S, Zhang B, Naito S, Hamaguchi H, Arakawa K: Apolipoprotein(a) phenotypes and serum lipoprotein(a) levels in maintenance hemodialysis patients with/without diabetes mellitus. Kidney Int 1993;44:1062–1070.

20 Okura Y, Saku K, Hirata K, Zhang B, Liu R, Ogahara S, Naito S, Kajiyama G, Arakawo K: Serum lipoprotein(a) levels in maintenance hemodialysis patients. Nephron 1993; 65:46–50.

21 Tschope W, Koch M, Thomas B, Ritz E, German Study Group Diabetes and Uremia: Serum lipids predict cardiac death in diabetic patients on maintenance hemodialysis: Results of a prospective study. Nephron 1993;64:354–358.

22 D'Elia JA, Weinrauch LA, Gleason RE, de Silva RA, Nestro R: Preliminary screening of the relationship of serum lipids to screening of chronic dialysis patients. Renal Fail 1993; 15:203–209.

23 Cressman MD, Abbound D, O'neil J, Hoff HF: Lp-(a) and premature mortality during hemodialysis treatment. Chem Phys Lipids 1994;67/68:419–427.

24 James TN: Morphologic characteristics and functional significance of focal fibromuscular dysplasia of small coronary arteries. Am J Cardiol 1990;65:12G–22G.

25 Rostand SG, Kirk KA, Rutsky EA: The epidemiology of coronary artery disease in patients on maintenance hemodialysis: Implications for management; in Wizemann V, Kramer W, Schütterle G (eds): The Heart in End-Stage Renal Failure. Contrib Nephrol. Basel, Karger, 1986, vol 52, pp 34–41.

26 Zoneraich S: Unravelling the conundrums of the diabetic heart diagnosed in 1876: Prelude to genetics. Can J Cardiol 1994;10:945–950.

27 Amann K, Wiest G, Zimmer G, Gretz N, Ritz E, Mall G: Reduced capillary density in the myocardium of uremic rats: A stereological study. Kidney Int 1992;42:1079–1085.

28 Raine AEG, Seymour A-ML, Roberts AFC, Radda GK, Ledingham JGG: Impairment of cardiac function and energetics in experimental renal failure. J Clin Invest 1993;92: 2934–2940.

29 Massry SG, Smogorzewski M: Mechanisms through which parathyroid hormone mediates its deleterious effects on organ function in uremia. Semin Nephrol 1994;14: 219–231.

30 Foley RN, Parfrey PS, Harnett JD, Kent GM, Hu L, Murray DC, Barre PE: Hypocalcemia, morbidity and mortality in end-stage renal disease. Am J Nephrol, in press.

31 Lacour B, Basile C, Drüeke T, Funck-Brentano JL: Parathyroid function and lipid metabolism in the rat. Miner Electrolyte Metab 1982;7:157–165.

32 Wizemann V, Kaufmann J, Kramer W: Effect of erythropoietin on ischemia tolerance in anemic hemodialysis patients with confirmed coronary artery disease. Nephron 1992; 62:161–165.

Blood Purification

Blood Purif 1996;14:327–333

Factors Affecting Renal Allograft Survival in African Americans

Robert S. Gaston

Department of Medicine, Division of Nephrology, and Department of Surgery, Division of Transplantation, University of Alabama at Birmingham, Birmingham, Ala., USA

Key Words

Kidney transplantation, African Americans
Socioeconomics, African Americans
HLA matching
Immunosuppression
Ciclosporin
Compliance, African Americans

Abstract

African Americans are more likely to develop end-stage renal disease than other racial groups. Although transplantation is optimal therapy for most end-stage renal disease patients, many potential black recipients do not have ready access to cadaveric kidneys. Following transplantation, blacks are at increased risk of allograft loss as a result of the interaction of multiple immunologic and nonimmunologic factors.

Because of changing trends in incidence and management of end-stage renal disease (ESRD), minority issues have assumed greater significance in recent years and generated substantial controversy. Due to multiple poorly characterized physiologic and socioeconomic factors, ESRD in the United States occurs with disproportionate frequency among blacks: while 12% of the general population is African American, 34% of the ESRD population is black [1]. In Alabama, African Americans make up 25% of the general population, but 67% of those with ESRD [2]. Although many nephrologists consider transplantation to be optimal therapy for chronic renal failure, blacks are less likely than other racial groups to receive transplants [3–7]. Finally, once transplanted, African Americans appear to be at increased risk of allograft loss relative to other racial groups, regardless of donor source or HLA match [8, 9]. While recognizing that these issues are interrelated and significantly influence the overall management of African Americans with kidney disease, this review will focus on specific factors which appear to adversely impact the outcome of transplantation in black recipients.

Race as a Risk Factor in Renal Transplantation

Since the publication of the landmark paper by Opelz, Mickey, and Terasaki [see ref. 11] in 1977, evidence has accumulated in both single- and multicenter studies that renal

KARGER

E-Mail karger@karger.ch
Fax + 41 61 306 12 34
http://www.karger.ch

0253–5068/96/0144–0327$10.00/0

Robert S. Gaston, MD
University of Alabama at Birmingham
Division of Nephrology, 625 THT
Birmingham, AL 35294 (USA)

transplantation is less successful in blacks than in whites [8, 10–12]. A decrement in graft survival for black recipients is evident within the first few months following transplantation and persists throughout subsequent intervals [8, 13]. Graft survival at 1 year is 4–20% lower for black recipients of comparably mismatched cadaveric and living-donor transplants [8, 10]. Even among those African Americans receiving completely matched cadaveric allografts, reduced graft survival at 1 year (89 vs. 81%) is well documented [8, 9]. Long-term outcomes are correspondingly diminished in blacks, with reduced graft survival at 3 and 5 years and a 40–50% reduction in half-life beyond 1 year [8, 13]. The half-life is, in fact, shorter for black recipients of living-related donor kidneys than for white recipients of cadaveric kidneys (8.2 vs. 7.9 years) [13].

Although the data are unambiguous, their implications are less straightforward: are African Americans at greater risk because of race and its corresponding genetics, or is race a proxy for some other negative influence? Butkus et al. [14] contend that when risk factors such as degree of HLA matching and socioeconomic status are removed from consideration, race exerts no independent effect on outcome. However, in their study of 57 black patients, 84% wre poorly matched, and 67% were in the lowest socioeconomic group, making it difficult to detect differences among additional contributing factors. Multivariate analysis of stratified data from the University of California at Los Angeles Registry found that, after adjusting for the effects of transplant center, donor race, recipient age, and HLA match, black recipients still had significantly reduced allograft survival relative to whites [15]. It seems likely that reduced graft survival in blacks is the result of the interaction of several adverse variables, of which some may be directly linked to race while others are not.

Immunologic Factors Affecting Allograft Survival in African Americans

A substantial body of knowledge indicates that black recipients are at increased risk of immunologic allograft loss. Transplanted African Americans are more likely to experience acute rejection than are recipients of other ethnic backgrounds [16]. In the United States, a black ESRD patient is less likely to have a suitable living donor, and more often requires cadaveric transplantion. Since cadaveric donors are drawn from the general population (predominantly white) and since there is significant racial disparity in HLA antigen expression, blacks are more likely to receive poorly matched transplants [17–19]. Although some consider poor matching to be the critical determinant of poorer outcomes for blacks [14], the contribution of HLA to racial differences in graft survival is more complex. Major histocompatibility complex antigens are less well characterized in African Americans than in Caucasians, and the correlation of functional immune responses, such as the mixed lymphocyte reaction, with HLA matching is stronger in whites than in blacks [20–22]. Clinically, despite improved matching, blacks may not demonstrate improved outcomes, even when receiving HLA-identical cadaveric allografts [9, 18, 23]. Recent technical advances in histocompatibility testing have improved the accuracy of tissue typing in blacks. Nonetheless, racial disparities between donor (predominantly white) and recipient (disproportionately black) populations obligate that any algorithm designed to increase the degree of HLA matching will produce the untoward effect of shunting kidneys away from black recipients [4, 5, 7]. Recognizing this dilemma, recent proposals have emphasized broader categories of matching which improve access of black candidates to cadaveric kidneys and may preserve the beneficial impact of better matching on outcomes in other racial groups [7, 24].

Apart from major histocompatibility complex related issues, other nonspecific immunologic factors may increase the risk for black Americans. Kerman et al. [25] noted that in a battery of immunologic tests (mixed lymphocyte reaction, T helper:T suppressor ratios, spontaneous blastogenesis) blacks were more likely than whites to be strong responders [25]; the outcome correlated with the overall immune response more than with the HLA match. In another study [26], these same authors found black recipients of blood transfusions more likely to respond with substantial anti-HLA antibody formation than similarly transfused whites.

Other evidence of enhanced immunologic responses in African Americans is to be found in a series of clinical observations indicating that black patients may benefit from more aggressive immunosuppression. Induction therapy, with both polyclonal and monoclonal antibodies, enhances outcomes in black recipients who also appear to be more resistant than whites to developing complications such as opportunistic infections [18, 27]. Hricik et al. [28] have found black recipients of cadaveric allografts to be more likely to experience acute rejection when discontinuing corticosteroid therapy than a comparable cohort of white recipients. Very recently, racial differences in response to a new immunosuppressant (mycophenolate mofetil) were noted during a multicenter, randomized trial [29]: higher doses (3 vs. 2 g) seemed necessary to achieve a beneficial therapeutic response in black recipients.

Nonimmunologic Factors Affecting Allograft Survival in African Americans

Given that matching does not explain the impact of race on transplant outcome and that conferring the attribute of immunologic hyperresponsiveness to blacks may be intellectually unsatisfying, some have emphasized the role of nonimmunologic factors in reducing graft survival for African Americans. As early as 1982, it was recognized that blacks were more likely to receive transplants at centers with suboptimal results [12, 30]. However, one can equally contend that these centers have worse results because they transplant more African Americans. In a recent review, Gjertson [31] analyzed outcomes by race among four graded categories of centers, ranging from those with suboptimal results (grade I) to those with excellent overall graft survival (grade IV). Grade I centers transplanted fewer white patients and slightly more African Americans than the remaining grades. However, among all four grades of centers, blacks demonstrated reduced half-lives relative to whites, making it difficult to associate inferior results in blacks with inferior care.

Although the incidence may be overestimated, hypertension persists as the most common cause of ESRD in African Americans [1, 32]. Oriol et al. [12] suggested that low graft survival might be a result of predisposition to vascular disease in blacks relative to whites. Clearly, hypertension following transplantation is predictive of increased risk of allograft loss [33, 34]. Recently, Cosio et al. [35] found poorly controlled posttransplant hypertension to be a stronger predictor of graft failure in blacks than immunologic factors, including HLA match and acute rejection episodes. However, in this study, it is conceivable that uncontrolled hypertension, rather than exert-

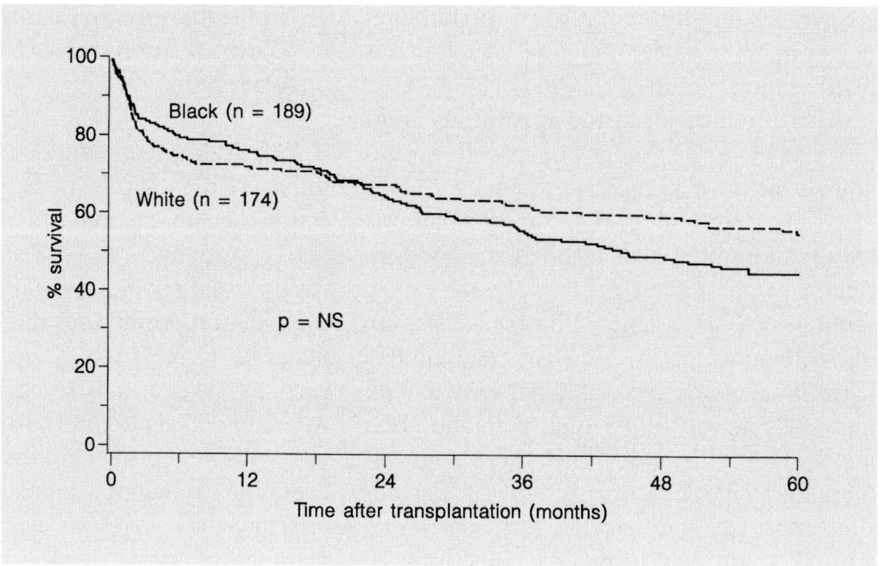

Fig. 1. Allograft survival for African American (—) and Caucasian (---) recipients of first cadaveric allografts at the University of Alabama at Birmingham Hospital during 1987–1990.

ing an independent effect, might be a marker of other important factors, such as compliance.

Other nonimmunologic influences thought to contribute to racial differences in short- and long-term outcome revolve around socioeconomic issues. Lower socioeconomic status is a predisposing factor for ESRD in African Americans [36, 37]. Likewise, economic disadvantage predicts poorer transplant outcomes [14, 38]. Butkus et al. [14] used insurance coverage at the time of transplantation as a proxy for socioeconomic status. Those patients without private insurance, who were more often African Americans, were at increased risk of allograft loss. Kalil et al. [38] found inadequate family income levels to be strongly associated with return to dialysis. The link between socioeconomic status and allograft failure may be noncompliance with medical regimens [38–40]. There are strong correlations among socioeconomic status, educational background, and medical compliance. Schweizer et al. [40] found noncompliance with medications and office visits to be a significant predictor of graft loss and to occur more often in blacks than in whites; however, after correcting for socioeconomic status, noncompliance occurred with an equal frequency among races. Likewise, although noncompliance influenced the risk of graft loss, insurance status rather than race was more closely associated with both adverse events in the Mississippi analysis [14].

Integrating Immunologic and Nonimmunologic Causes of Graft Loss

As in most aspects of medicine, clinical results in transplantation likely reflect the interaction of multiple influences that never truly exert an independent effect. In our experience at the University of Alabama at Birmingham, there appear to be both early and late phases of increased allograft loss among black recipients. Before 1987, African Americans patients were more likely than Caucasians to experience early acute rejection episodes, with a correspondingly increased risk of allograft loss during the first 3 months following transplantation [10, 18]. The use of antibody induction (with polyclonal or monoclonal antibody preparations) abolished these early differences in primary recipients, with similar allograft survival achieved for both whites and blacks at 1 year (fig. 1) [18]. We interpret these results as indicating that enhanced immunologic responsiveness in African American recipients can be suppressed by aggressive immunosuppression, particularly during the early posttransplant period.

However, as can be seen from figure 1, there is a second phase of increased risk for black recipients which persists despite quadruple therapy. Decay in graft survival occurs over time among all recipients, but is more pronounced in African Americans after the first 2 years. The cause of this long-term increased risk for blacks is more difficult to analyze, but may represent the interplay of several factors. If noncompliance occurs more commonly among the economically disadvantaged (who are disproportionately African American), it seems likely that the presence of immunologic hyperresponsiveness among black recipients (whether due to poorer HLA matching or innate immunologic reactivity) may enhance the risk for graft loss. A Caucasian recipient demonstrating similar noncompliance may fare better than his African American counterpart.

This hypothesis has been tested in our own experience at the University of Alabama at Birmingham [41]. Due to financial constraints imposed by discontinuation of Medicare payment for immunosuppressive drugs at 1 year, 42 patients with excellent allograft function at 1 year were tapered off ciclosporin over several months. Among 19 white recipients, there were no significant adverse effects. However, 13 of 23 black recipients experienced acute rejection after discontinuing ciclosporin, and 7 lost their grafts as a consequence. 'Iatrogenic noncompliance' was a high-risk proposition for these African Americans, presumably reflecting the adverse interaction of enhanced immunologic responsiveness and disadvantaged socioeconomic status.

Conclusions

The optimal approach to attenuating racial differences in allograft survival would be to reduce the incidence of ESRD in the black community. Although enormous efforts are under way to better define and treat the pathogenetic elements involved, socioeconomic obstacles may prove more refractory; it seems likely that the ESRD population will remain disproportionately black. It appears that the nonimmunologic factors predisposing black recipients to ESRD are in many ways similar to those that promulgate allograft loss (hypertension, medication compliance, access to health care). The nature of enhanced immunologic responsiveness in African Americans must be better characterized and its impact reduced by further improvements in immunosuppressive therapy. Accordingly, allocation algorithms designed to enhance HLA matching for black and white recipients must acknowledge and address impact on issues of access [4, 42]. Recognizing and eliminating racial disparities in transplantation remains a significant challenge for the nephrology community.

References

1 United States Renal Data System. 1994 Annual Data Report IV. Incidence and causes of treated ESRD. Am J Kidney Dis 1994;24(suppl): 48–56.
2 Network 8. 1993 Annual Data Report. 1994.
3 Eggers PW: Effect of transplantation on the Medicare End-Stage Renal Disease Program. N Engl J Med 1988;318:223–229.
4 Gaston RS, Ayres I, Dooley LG, Diethelm AG: Racial equity in renal transplantation: The disparate impact of HLA-based allocation. JAMA 1993;270:1352–1356.
5 Held PJ, Kahan BD, Hunsicker LG, Liska D, Wolfe RA, Port FK, Gaylin DS, Garcia JR, Agodoa LYC, Krakauer H: The impact of HLA mismatches on the survival of first cadaveric kidney transplants. N Engl J Med 1994;331:765–770.
6 Sanfilippo F: HLA matching in renal transplantation. N Engl J Med 1994;331:803–805.
7 Takemoto S, Terasaki PI, Gjertson DW, Cecka JM: Equitable allocation of HLA-compatible kidneys for local pools and for minorities. N Engl J Med 1994;331:760–764.
8 Cecka JM, Terasaki PI: The UNOS Scientific Renal Transplant Registry; in Terasaki PI, Cecka JM (eds): Clinical Transplants 1993. Los Angeles, UCLA Tissue Typing Laboratory, 1993, pp 1–18.
9 Takemoto S, Terasaki PI, Cecka JM, Cho YW, Gjertson DW: Survival of nationally shared, HLA-matched kidney transplants from cadaveric donors. N Engl J Med 1992;327:834–839.
10 Barger BO, Hudson SL, Shroyer TW, Deierhoi MH, Barber WH, Curtis JJ, Julian BA, Luke RG, Diethelm AG: Influence of race on renal allograft survival in the pre- and postciclosporine era; in Terasaki PI (ed): Clinical Transplants 1987. Los Angeles, UCLA Tissue Typing Laboratory, 1987, pp 217–233.
11 Opelz G, Mickey MR, Terasaki PI: Influence of race on kidney transplant survival. Transplant Proc 1977;9:137–142.
12 Oriol R, LePendu J, Chun C: Influence of the original disease, race, and center on the outcome of kidney transplantation. Transplantation 1982;33:22–26.
13 Yuge J, Burgos D: Long-term kidney graft survival; in Terasaki PI, Cecka JM (eds): Clinical Transplants 1992. Los Angeles, UCLA Tissue Typing Laboratory, 1992, pp 319–331.
14 Butkus DE, Meydrech EF, Raju SS: Racial differences in the survival of cadaveric renal allografts: Overriding effects of HLA matching and socioeconomic factors. N Engl J Med 1992;327:840–845.
15 Zhou YC, Cecka JM, Terasaki PI: Effect of race on kidney transplants; in Terasaki PI (eds): Clinical Transplants 1990. Los Angeles, UCLA Tissue Typing Laboratory, 1990, pp 447–459.
16 Koyama H, Cecka JM: Race effects; in Terasaki PI, Cecka JM (eds): Clinical Transplants 1991. Los Angeles, UCLA Tissue Typing Laboratory, 1991, pp 269–280.
17 Lazda VA, Blaesing ME: Is allocation of kidneys on basis of HLA match equitable in multiracial populations? Transplant Proc 1989;21: 1415–1416.
18 Gaston RS, Hudson SL, Deierhoi MH, Barber WH, Laskow DA, Julian BA, Curtis JJ, Barger BO, Shroyer TW, Diethelm AG: Improved survival of primary cadaveric renal allografts in blacks with quadruple immunosuppression. Transplantation 1992;53:103–109.
19 Leffell MS, Steinberg AG, Bias WB, Machan CH, Zachary AA: The distribution of HLA antigens and phenotypes among donors and patients in the UNOS Registry. Transplantation 1994;58:1119–1130.
20 Johnson AH, Rosen-Bronson S, Hurley CK: Heterogeneity of the HLA-D region in American blacks. Transplant Proc 1989;21:3872–3873.
21 Milford EL, Ratner L, Yunis E: Will transplant immunogenetics lead to better graft survival in blacks? Racial variability in the accuracy of tissue typing for organ donation: The Fourth American Workshop. Transplant Proc 1987;19(suppl 2):30–32.
22 Suciu-Foca N, Reed E, Rohowsky C, Lewison A, King DW: Influence of race on the predictability of mixed lymphocyte culture identity by HLA DR matching. Transplantation 1983; 35:35–39.
23 Opelz G, Pfarr E, Engelmann A, Keppel E: Kidney graft survival rates in black ciclosporin-treated patients. Transplant Proc 1989;21: 3918–3920.
24 Hudson SL, Shroyer TW, Deierhoi MH, Gaston RS, Diethelm AG: CREG Matching and Racial Equity: A Retrospective Look at Graft Survival in 1692 Cadaveric Renal Transplants at a Single Center (abstract). Pittsburgh, American Society of Histocompatibility and Immunogenetics, 1994.
25 Kerman RH, Kimball PM, Van Buren CT, Lewis RM, Kahan BD: Possible contribution of pretransplant immune responder status to renal allograft survival differences of black versus white recipients. Transplantation 1991;51:338–342.
26 Kerman RH, Kimball PM, Van Buren CT, Lewis RM, Cavazos D, Heydari A, Kahan BD: Influence of race on crossmatch outcome and recipient eligibility for transplantation. Transplantation 1992;53:64–67.
27 Butkus DE: Primary renal cadaveric allograft survival in blacks: Is there still a significant difference. Transplant Rev 1991;5:91–99.
28 Hricik DE, Whalen CC, Lautman J, Bartucci MR, Moir EJ, Mayes JT, Schulak JA: Withdrawal of steroids after renal transplantation: Clinical predictors of outcome. Transplantation 1992;53:41–45.
29 Neylan JF, Deierhoi MH: Dose-Dependent Prevention of Acute Renal Transplant Rejection in African Americans Receiving Mycophenolate Mofetil (abstract). Chicago, American Society of Transplant Physicians, 1995.
30 Perdue ST, Terasaki PI: Analysis of interracial variation in kidney transplant and patient survival. Transplantation 1982;34:75–77.

31 Gjertson DW: Center-dependent transplantation factors: An analysis of renal allografts reported to the UNOS Registry; in Terasaki PI, Cecka JM (eds): Clinical Transplants 1993. Los Angeles, UCLA Tissue Typing Laboratory, 1993, pp 445–468.
32 Schlessinger SD, Tankersley MR, Curtis JJ: Clinical documentation of end-stage renal disease due to hypertension. Am J Kidney Dis 1994;23: 655–660.
33 Curtis JJ: Hypertension and kidney transplantation. Am J Kidney Dis 1986;7:181–196.
34 Brazy PC, Pirsch JD, Belzer FO: Factors affecting renal allograft function in long-term recipients. Am J Kidney Dis 1992;19:558–566.
35 Cosio FG, Dillon JJ, Falkenhain ME, Tesi RJ, Henry ML, Elkhammas EA, Davies EA, Bumgardner GL, Ferguson RM: Racial differences in renal allograft survival: The role of systemic hypertension. Kidney Int 1995;47:1136–1141.
36 Rostand SG: US minority groups and end-stage renal disease: A disproportionate share. Am J Kidney Dis 1992;19:411–413.
37 Qualheim RE, Rostand SG, Kirk KA, Rutsky EA, Luke RG: Changing patterns of end-stage renal disease due to hypertension. Am J Kidney Dis 1991;18:336–343.
38 Kalil RSN, Heim-Duthoy KL, Kasiske BL: Patients with a low income have reduced renal allograft survival. Am J Kidney Dis 1992;20:63–69.
39 Didlake RH, Dreyfus K, Kerman RH, Van Buren CT, Kahan BD: Patient noncompliance: A major cause of large graft failure in ciclosporin-treated renal transplants. Transplant Proc 1988;20(suppl 3):63–69.
40 Schweizer RT, Rovelli M, Palmeri D, Vossler E, Hull D, Bartus S: Noncompliance in organ transplant recipients. Transplantation 1990;49: 374–377.
41 Sanders CE, Curtis JJ, Julian BA, Gaston RS, Jones PA, Laskow DA, Deierhoi MH, Barber WH, Diethelm AG: Tapering or discontinuing ciclosporin for financial reasons: A single center experience. Am J Kidney Dis 1993;21:9–15.
42 Gaston RS, Deierhoi MH, Ayres I: HLA matching in renal transplantation. N Engl J Med 1995;332:752–753.

Author Index Vol. 14, No. 4, 1996

Subject Index Vol. 14, No. 4, 1996